CRYSTAL HEALING

&

SACRED PLEASURE

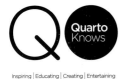

Brimming with creative inspiration, how-to projects, and useful information to enrich your everyday life, Quarto Knows is a favorite destination for those pursuing their interests and passions. Visit our site and dig deeper with our books into your area of interest: Quarto Creates, Quarto Cooks, Quarto Homes, Quarto Lives, Quarto Drives, Quarto Explores, Quarto Gifts, or Quarto Kids.

Inspiring | Educating | Creating | Entertaining

First Published in 2018 by Fair Winds Press, an imprint of The Quarto Group,
100 Cummings Center, Suite 265-D, Beverly, MA 01915, USA.
T (978) 282-9590 F (978) 283-2742 QuartoKnows.com

Fair Winds Press titles are also available at discount for retail, wholesale, promotional, and bulk purchase. For details, contact the Special Sales Manager by email at specialsales@quarto.com or by mail at The Quarto Group, Attn: Special Sales Manager, 401 Second Avenue North, Suite 310, Minneapolis, MN 55401, USA.

22 21 20 19 18   1 2 3 4 5

ISBN: 978-1-59233-818-4

Library of Congress Cataloging-in-Publication Data is available

Cover design, page design, and page layout: Tanya Jacobson, tanyasoffice.com
Photography Art Direction: Jennifer Sotelo
Lifestyle Photography: Rachel Cuccia
Still Photography: Kate Hollowell
Stylist: Dessislava Terzieva
Hair Stylist: Marisa Cuccia
Illustration: Ada Keesler @adagracee

Printed in China

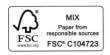

The information in this book is for educational purposes only. It is not intended to replace the advice of a physician or medical practitioner. Please see your health-care provider before beginning any new health program.

Chakrubs™ and The Original Crystal Sex Toy Company® are trademarks of Vanessa Cuccia.

CRYSTAL HEALING

&

SACRED PLEASURE

Awaken Your Sensual Energy Using Crystals and
Healing Rituals, One Chakra at a Time

VANESSA CUCCIA

founder of Chakrubs™

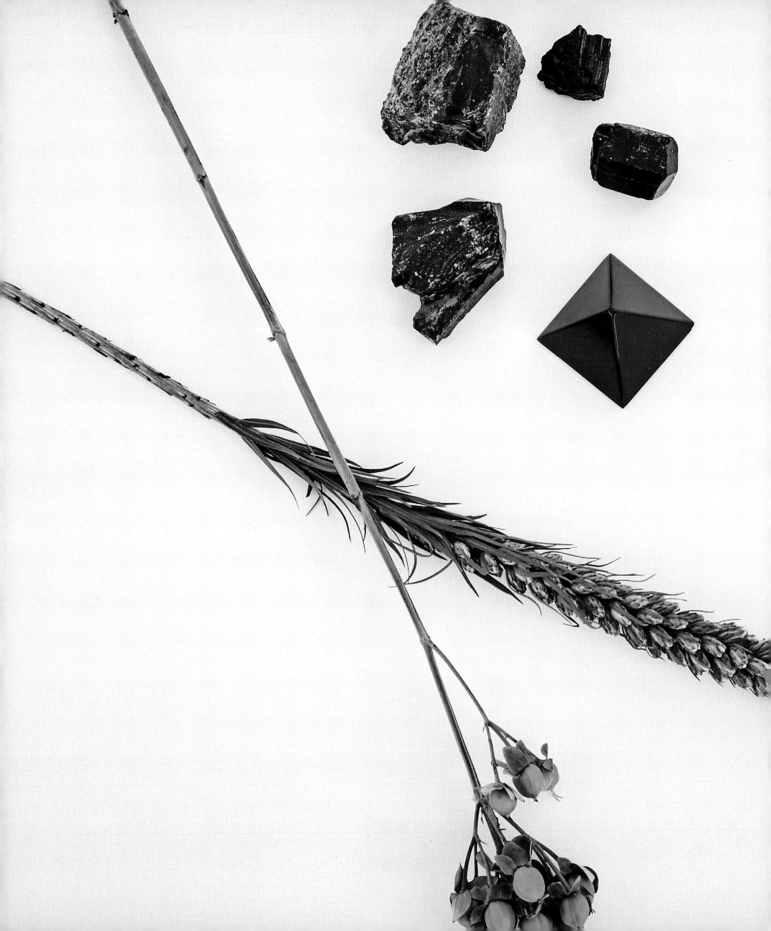

CONTENTS

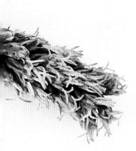

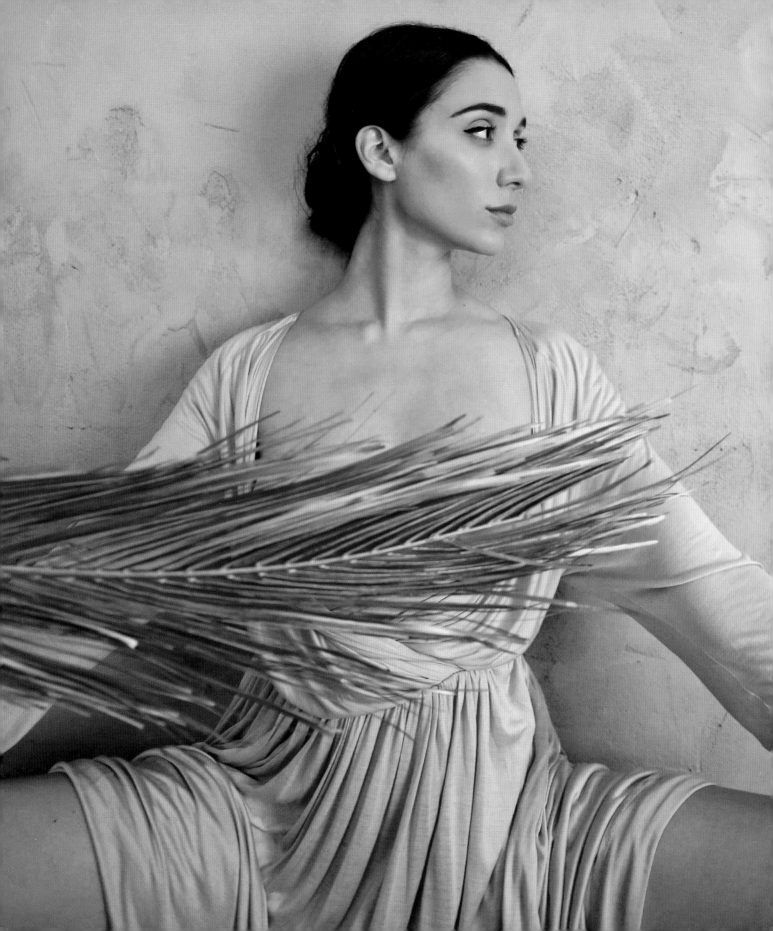

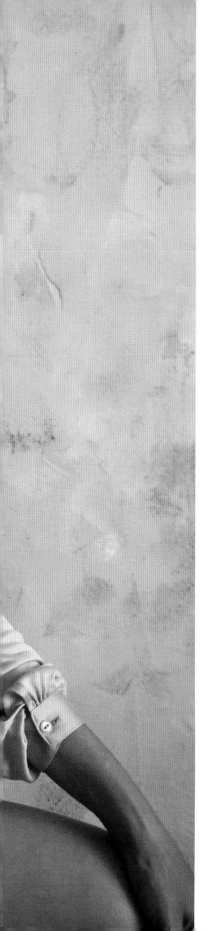

Preface

Crack open a seemingly ordinary geode, and you will discover a beautiful crystalline interior. This is you. Go beyond the aesthetics of a crystal, and you will unearth the potency of its energy. This is also you. It can be an intimidating task to uncover yourself, but that is only because deep within you lies great power. You hold massive potential: your body for ecstasy, your spirit for connection, and your heart for love.

This book will assist you on the path of accessing pleasure to awaken your purpose and empower your entire being. The use of crystals in this work serves two primary functions. One is to act as a support system and grounding element so that you know you are safe, secure, and protected as you explore your sexual, emotional, and spiritual well-being. The other is to act as conduits to your own higher realms of understanding. You see, you already hold the answers you seek inside of you; it's just about being open enough to integrate them into your daily life. Crystals themselves do not heal. Crystals aid your natural healing abilities by facilitating movement within your energetic system (otherwise known as your chakras).

We will begin this journey by addressing your current mindset. If you are open, you won't need any specific belief system to benefit from the practices contained in this book. You will learn how to use crystals to help sensitize yourself to the subtle energies of the universe. Whether or not you currently feel a connection to these forces, you will learn how to interact with and benefit from them for the purpose of self-realization. You will learn how crystals are formed and how to choose the appropriate ones for you. You will learn how to charge and cleanse your crystals in order to harness their countless benefits. This will be supplemented with information about your chakras and how they reveal themselves in different areas of your life. You will be given tools for keeping your chakra system healthy using crystal therapy and sensual exercises.

Many books on chakras only briefly touch upon the sexual potency of the chakra system. However, through my work as a provider of crystals dedicated to healing through sexual expression and self-love practices, I have discovered that when one is able to connect on any of these levels, one's sexual energy increases. It feels sexy to be connected to primal instincts (root chakra). It feels sexy to have a drive to relate to others (sacral chakra). It feels sexy to be empowered by the belief that you can manifest whatever you want (solar plexus chakra). It feels sexy to have an open heart and to give and receive love freely (heart chakra). It feels sexy to openly express creativity and ideas (throat chakra). It feels sexy to listens to your intuition (third eye chakra). It feels sexy to be connected to source energy (crown chakra). And feeling sexy is an empowered state of being. Sexy people radiate self-possession, curiosity, and compassion.

In a world that is becoming increasingly disconnected and de-sensitized, we need to reclaim what we crave most: intimacy and connection. It may seem that with all the apps for dating, hook-up culture, divorce rates, fewer marriages, and porn addictions, society is leaning toward a superficial reality based on technology. This may cause you to feel alone in your pursuit. I once felt this way too.

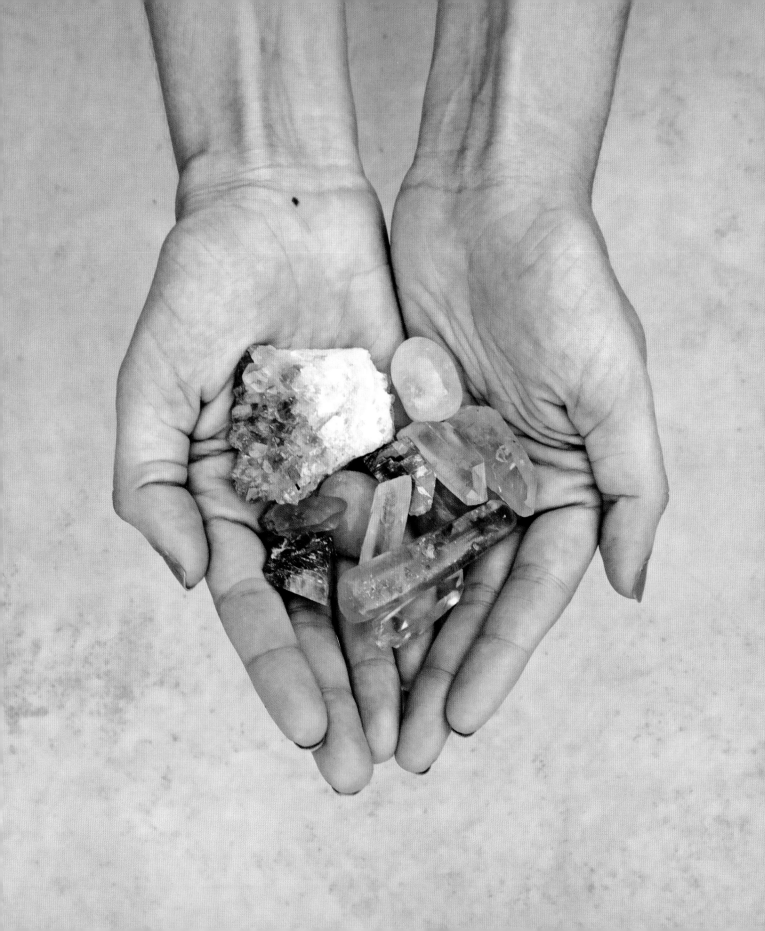

Since puberty, I felt alone in my ideals of connection, love, and sex. It seemed that among my peers, I was the outcast who wanted to wait until I truly felt in love to have sex. I always believed that my own sexuality would develop once I felt connected with another person. This perception was altered when I lost my virginity at the age of seventeen to a boyfriend who did not ask for my consent. This story is quite common. I continue to hear experiences at workshops from people who share it. When your first introduction to sex is not a positive one, it is usually difficult to release the feelings you may have repressed from those experiences, especially if you are young and still developing emotional intelligence. After my experience, I made the conscious decision to not feel as if I were a victim but rather to "fall in love" with my boyfriend, so that I could develop an inkling of that feeling I wanted. But after six years of this relationship, I finally realized that I was repressing my true feelings, that I was disassociating from my body during sex, and that pleasure (sex) was something I was giving but not fully receiving in return.

Perhaps what I had attempted to do was noble. After all, lying to myself through the years to shield myself from pain was the best tool I had to help me cope. But I picked up a new tool, finally, that would help change my life forever. On our way cross-country from New York to California to pursue careers in music, my boyfriend and I stopped at a crystal shop in Arizona. I was immediately drawn to the crystals, remembering cracking geodes with my family at the bluffs on Long Island when I was a child. This was part of my story I had forgotten. Admiring the beauty and discovering the majesty of the earth used to be something I loved. At this little shop, each crystal had attributes ascribed to it on slips of paper. One represented creativity; another, guidance. I purchased these stones and took them with me on my journey. Just like that, I had a new tool. Self-reflection.

As I grew older, I knew that if I wanted to be happy in my life, I needed to make a change. I needed to reclaim the pleasure of my body and connect to myself so that I would feel empowered to set boundaries. I needed to tune into what I had been ignoring in my relationship—my sense of self and my connection to spirit. I thought back to the views on sexuality I had before I'd met my boyfriend and decided that even if my attitudes of sexuality hadn't been popular among my peers, I owed it to myself to give them the attention they deserved and to accept who I was.

I dedicated myself to expanding my knowledge of crystals and energy healing and would eventually earn certifications in Reiki. I took a part-time job at an adult shop to educate myself on sexuality and be around sex-positive people who could help me to better understand the sexual desires I hadn't been addressing. I learned about every sex toy on the market, but I knew that I needed more knowledge than how to have a great orgasm. I needed to heal myself of the sexual and emotional traumas I had endured, re-inhabit my body, and keep my heart open to love. It was the combination of these needs that led me to create the Chakrub, a crystal specially designed for intimate use. I founded Chakrubs, The Original Crystal Sex Toy Company, because I felt that this method for healing myself could also benefit others. As I continue to learn and share many wonderful stories of self-healing through crystal energy, this modality is becoming better recognized around the world.

Chakrubs has since been featured in top magazines, museums (on display as interactive sculptures), digital publications, five-star hotels, and on late-night talk shows and daytime television. The products are currently in more than 30 stores worldwide, and the message behind them continues to spread beyond.

The most gratifying aspect of my work are the testimonials I receive from customers. They share stories of overcoming the fear of being touched, of becoming more comfortable in their bodies, and of igniting passion back into 35-year-long relationships, among others. The more I read, the more I realized that I was not alone at all, and that there are thousands—if not millions—of people who have the same inclination to honor their sexuality as sacred. To those of you who wish to celebrate your own personal desires and honor your sacredness, I offer you this first edition.

Throughout this book we will utilize the ancient wisdom of the body's energy system and crystals, along with modern application for self-love practices. Each ritual uses crystals as support systems, energy enhancers, and as an aspect of pleasure. I urge you to get excited about exploring yourself, and I welcome you to your individual path of self-discovery.

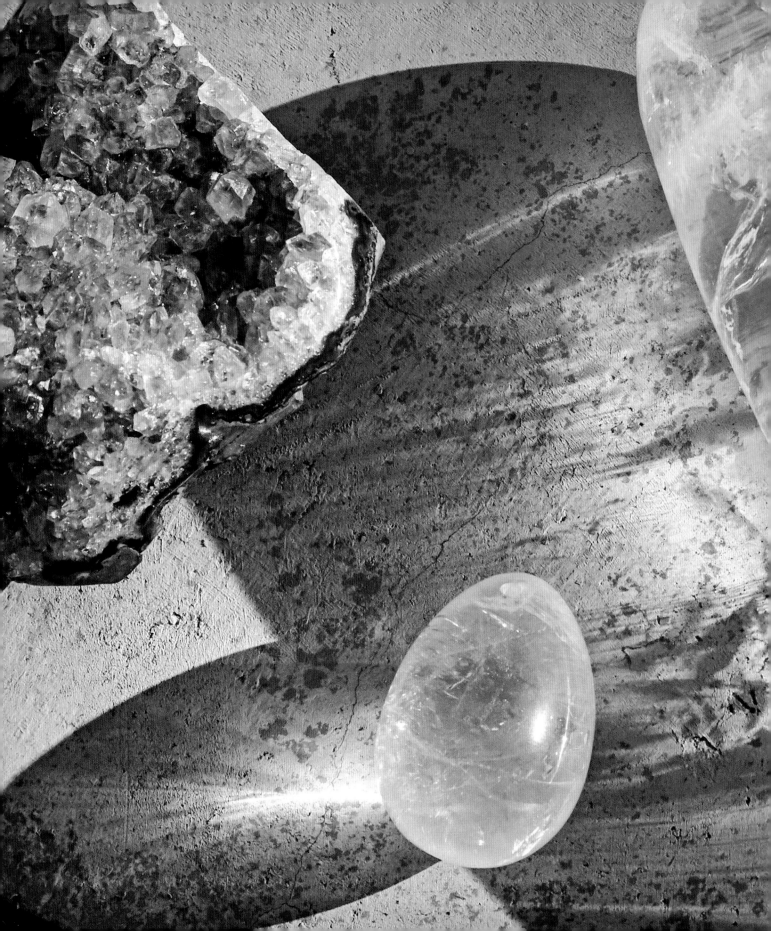

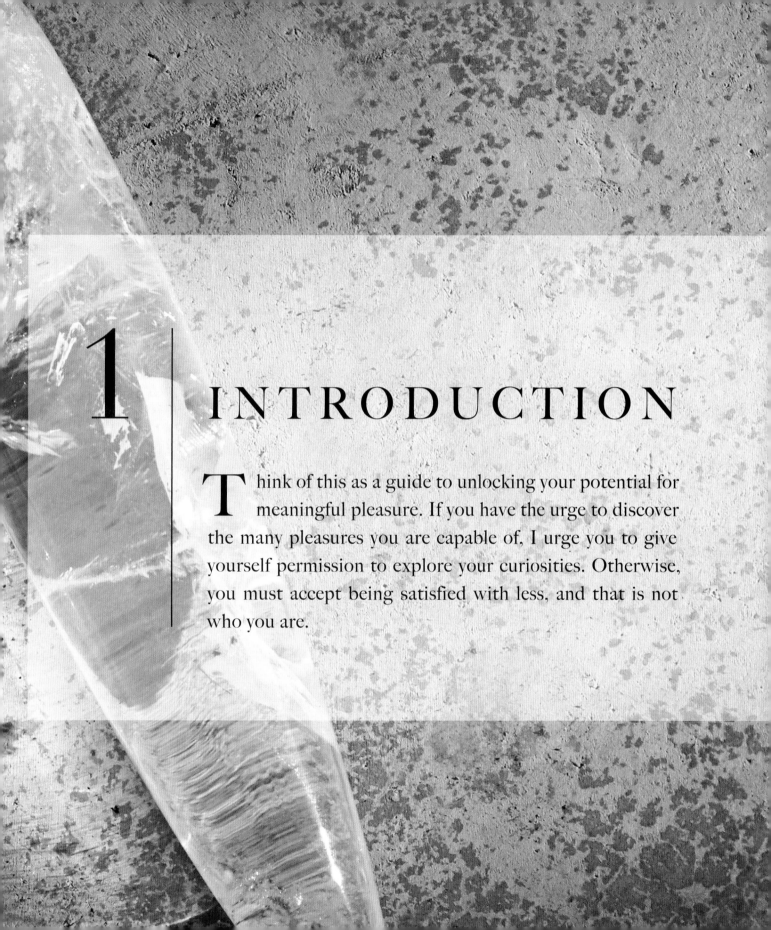

1 | INTRODUCTION

Think of this as a guide to unlocking your potential for meaningful pleasure. If you have the urge to discover the many pleasures you are capable of, I urge you to give yourself permission to explore your curiosities. Otherwise, you must accept being satisfied with less, and that is not who you are.

“*YOUR BODY AND THE EARTH
ARE CONDUITS
FOR THE DIVINE.*”

How you treat and experience your body creates energy that circulates through every area of your life. When you become an ally with your body, learn to listen to its needs, and nourish it through mindful affection, you create a sense of self-worth that permeates through your aura. Sensuality is an important part of this. Sexual energy vitalizes us when we learn to channel it and understand it as a tool. Sacred pleasure is the act of placing awareness on the spiritual significance of sensuous satisfaction and expression.

Being awakened sexually gives you the ability to feel orgasmic sensibility anytime you want. It's like muscle memory. You can call upon it when you want to feel more creative, more grateful, or more alert. It is yours, and you can cultivate it and direct it toward what you choose.

Prioritizing pleasure is empowering. People sense and respond positively when they feel you are rooted in pleasure. We normally think about communicating with others in terms of having a conversation, but speaking itself encompasses just a small percentage of communication. It also includes body language, facial expressions, and tone of voice. These elements of communication are all altered by our internal energy. We all know the feeling of walking into a room and noticing that something feels "off," or of being drawn to people who have a vibrant presence. Tense bodies give off tense energy. Relaxed bodies give off relaxed energy. We are all communicating with each others' energies on a constant basis, whether we recognize it or not.

It's important to learn to communicate with *yourself*, too. My sexual awakening came as a result of respecting my own boundaries. Learning to say "no" to sexual experiences and people I didn't want was liberating for me. This book will help you explore your sexuality so you can get to know yourself at different levels: your body, your energy, and your emotions. Through this process, you will find what it means to be sexually awakened for *you*.

You Are Magic Incarnate

Your divinity can be found in your humanity. The power you seek doesn't come from some outside source. But you, like many people, may be in a constant state of waiting, hoping for some kind of permission or initiation into a world beyond your knowledge. You seek it because you know it exists; it was ingrained into your subconsciousness as a child, through fairy tales and fables. Your youthful imagination allowed you to tap into something special and unseen, but over time you gave up believing. The problem is that many of us haven't matured our definitions of words like *magic*. We think it has to be grand and dramatic, like a fantasy.

But the truth is, you have the choice to open yourself up to cathartic experiences—to "magic"—at any time. Your body and the earth are conduits for the divine. When you look deeply inward, you are also looking at the beyond. Understanding divine concepts happens when you understand yourself. You—your body, what you have become numb to and deemed normal—are magic incarnate. Recognizing your own inherent power and learning to channel that power into something useful will help open your mind to experiencing more profound and at times even mystical, experiences. You can transform yourself, heal yourself, and embrace love for yourself and others. Everything—you, your thoughts, your body, your soul—is energy. Learning to work within energy systems is how you can create an empowered approach to life.

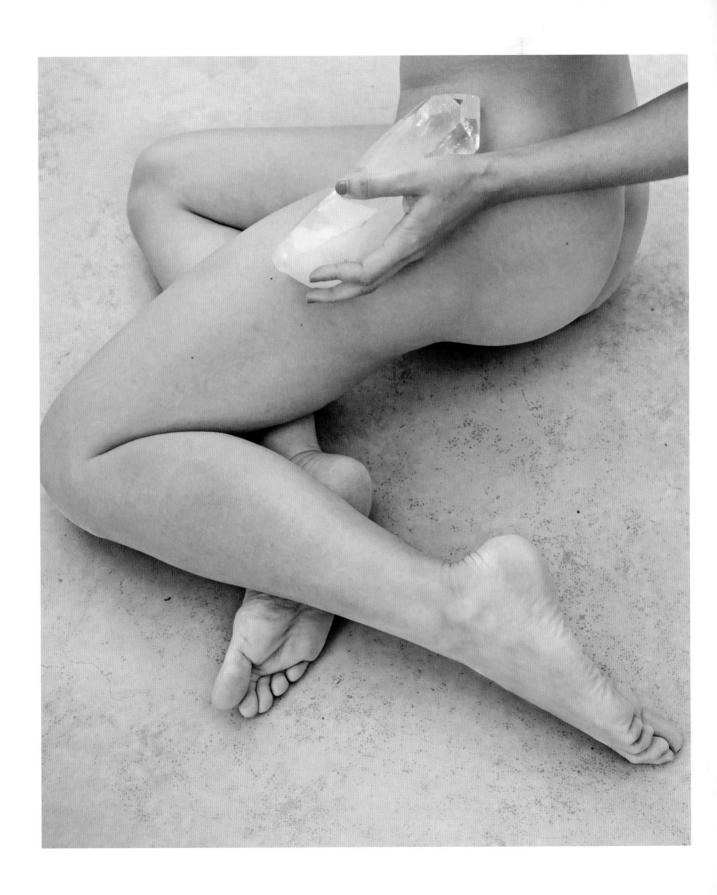

The Magic of Love and Sex

As children, just as we stop believing in otherworldly entities, we're introduced to a new kind of magic, one that even our parents still subscribe to: love and sex. We start seeing it everywhere. It's a new promised land filled with the hidden treasures of romance, eroticism, sexual chemistry, devotion, and the like. By the time puberty sets in, we're no longer preoccupied with disappointments about the Tooth Fairy not being real. We become focused on how to touch and be touched, how to fall in love, and how to feel. It's magic in a more acceptable, more "grown-up" form. We imagine that the first time we have sex will be a romantically epic, ecstatic experience. We think that orgasms are the end-all be-all, and sharing them with someone is cause for celebration. Then somewhere along the line, we experience more disappointment: With love comes sorrow, and orgasms only last seconds at a time. You begin to wonder, is this all there is to life?

This is a time for reflection, a time to dig deeper.

Being an adult doesn't mean giving up what you once believed in order to get in touch with "reality;" it means finding the deeper truth and holding onto your childlike curiosity. Once you reassess what magic is to you, you'll be able to recognize it in its true form. And it's everywhere. You can start by looking within yourself.

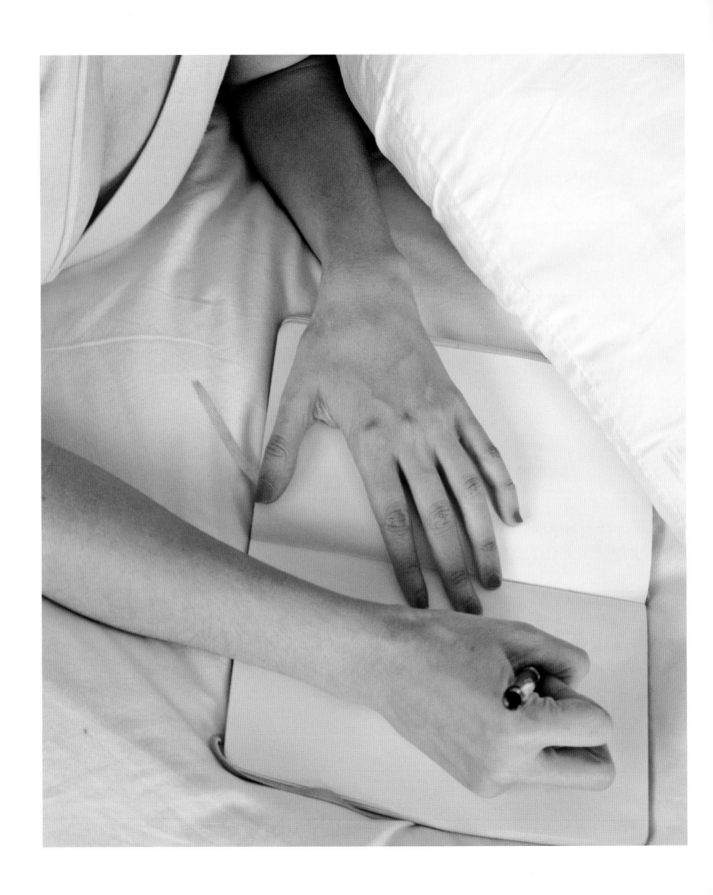

STAY GROUNDED
AND AWARE OF
YOUR FEELINGS
AND EXPERIENCES
BY KEEPING A
PERSONAL JOURNAL.

Remain Grounded

Some people are more sensitive to subtle energies than others. Working with focused intention and crystals can induce states of intense emotions, cause visions, increase awareness, and heighten sensitivity of touch, hearing, and the other senses. Many times, when people begin working with mystical modalities such as crystals, they open up a channel of awareness that can be very exciting.

You may find it helpful, when starting with crystal and chakra healing, to keep a journal to write down what sensations, thoughts, or visions come through after a session of meditation or ritual. Journaling enables you to observe what changes occur over time, or how things vary from each crystal or chakra center to another. Over time, you may receive messages of guidance so profound that you will be eager to share them with everyone. I encourage you to view your spiritual experiences as personal and intimate. Others can only understand on a deeper level if they have shared similar experiences. It's natural to want to share the joy of your newly found discoveries, but I suggest spending time with your discoveries alone. This way, they may become rooted in your subconscious as your own cherished and unique experiences.

As you become acquainted with the practices in this book, let yourself be free of self-judgment in order to focus on feeling. But remain curious and open by refusing to adopt an "I know all the answers" attitude. Deep within, you do know the answers. But it is part of being human to not know, to forget. True enlightenment is not something that can be explained: It has to be experienced.

One of the reasons I love crystals is their natural grounding element. Stones that aid in spiritual awakening are still grounding; they serve as a reminder to anchor ourselves in our bodies and remain footed on the earth while we explore other realms of consciousness. Deepen your understanding and hone your intuition by questioning. You don't have to doubt yourself or your feelings, but remain open and hold on to childlike curiosity. When you feel like you know it all, you stop learning, and there will always be something to learn.

And If You're a Skeptic, Welcome

Many people do *not* feel sensitive to subtle energy and may battle with thoughts that are self-defeating. However, if you were open enough to pick up this book, you are open enough to benefit from the therapeutic effects of working with crystals for self-love. It is also why self-pleasure is a recurring part of many of the following exercises. Arousal can be easily understood as energy, and recognizing this truth is the first step to directing that energy. If you have trouble believing in the metaphysical properties of the various crystals listed in this book, try thinking of them as physical representations of their listed benefits.

My goal is to help you empower yourself by encouraging you to accept and learn to find the value in all things—any thought or feeling, for example—that arises in you. The practices on the following pages serve as a guide for you to observe yourself and create more loving awareness through what you experience. Make whatever modifications you need to allow the experience to feel truer to you. Redefine the more "new-age" ideas in ways that resonate with you, if it will help remove resistance to receiving the advantages of this work.

Recently, I met with a woman who was well-known for being an atheist and general "skeptic." She hadn't expected us to get along, but we quickly dropped the walls that typically emerge when people like us meet for the first time. I commended her for raising questions about religion and spiritual topics. In the same way that she disowned the religion taught to her by her parents, I had disowned what I had been brought up to believe—that sex wasn't that big a deal, and that in this world what you see is what you get. For me, it made more sense to believe that sexuality ran deeper than orgasm and that we can feel subtle energy when we sensitize ourselves to it. This acknowledgment woke me out of a deep sleep state and directed me on a path that I am more than content to be on.

She was prepared to tell me that my proclivities toward crystal healing were ridiculous. What I saw was that through her need to deny "spiritual" concepts, she was denying herself something she deeply desired but was not willing to admit. Her identity had been created around calling "bullshit" on every new-agey spiritual concept. Instead, I wanted to appeal to her through the logical side of crystal healing.

I explained that even if she didn't feel the energetic vibrations emanating from the crystals, she could use them as reminders of what she felt she needed emotional support with. I learned that she had gone through a bad breakup a year before and had sworn off men ever since. Hesitantly,

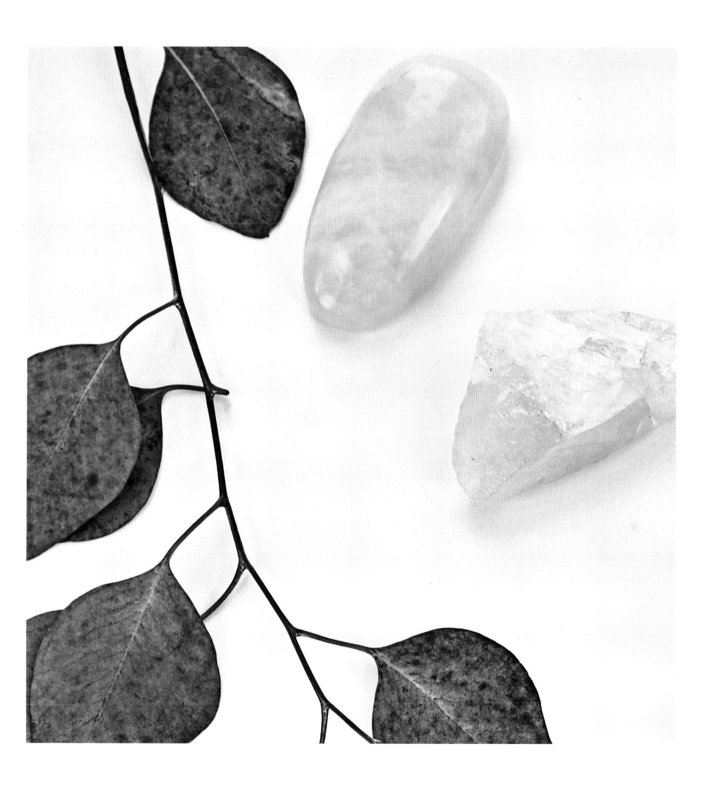

ROSE QUARTZ IS A TALISMAN FOR RELATIONSHIPS. IT CAN BE USED AS A POWERFUL APHRODISIAC AND HELP ONE GET IN TOUCH WITH THEIR SENSUALITY.

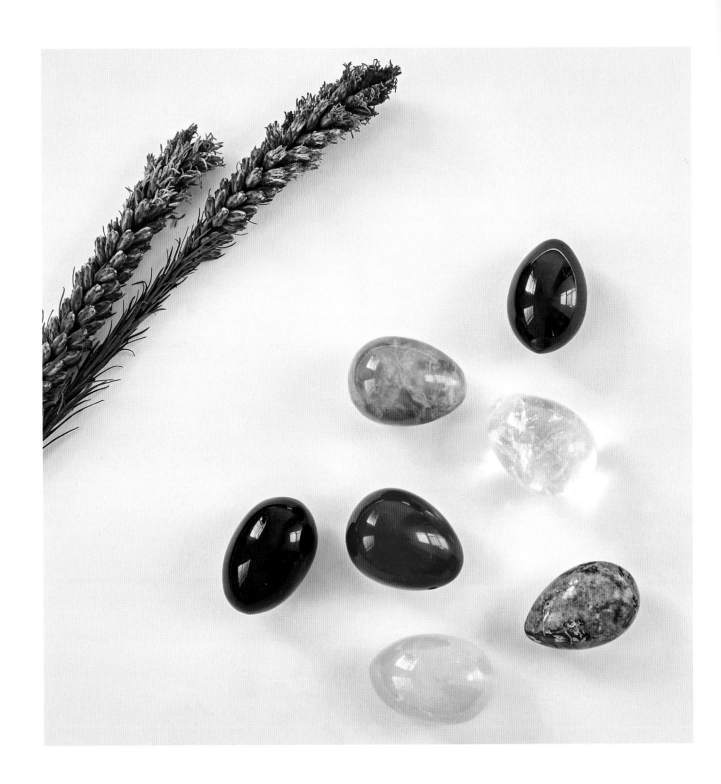

PAY ATTENTION TO THE SYMBOLS, SHAPES, AND COLORS THAT RESONATE FOR YOU.
THIS IS THE LANGUAGE OF YOUR SUBCONSCIOUS.

she told me that she wanted to feel love again but was afraid. I gave her a rose quartz stone and asked her to keep it in her purse. Every time she touched or saw the crystal, she was going to be reminded of what it stood for: being open and unafraid to love and be loved.

She didn't need to feel the physical sensations that some people feel when they use crystals; she needed the mental reminders of her intention to strengthen her intentions. A year later, she was in a relationship with someone for eight months.

To benefit from any type of non-traditional healing, you need to find the way that resonates with you. Your love and your story of healing will not look exactly like anyone else's, because you are the only one who has your exact experiences and perceptions. All you need to do is find the understanding that brings the most resonance. If it feels right for you to approach crystal therapy with a more logical mind at first, do this. All I ask is that you be open enough to experience what you need to experience, to stick with it, and to see the value in whatever comes up for you in the process.

Remove Resistance by Valuing Your Subconscious Language of Symbols

A great way to view the therapeutic practices offered in this book, especially if you consider yourself a skeptic, is through understanding the language of your subconscious. Your subconscious speaks through symbols, which is why in dreams you'll often conjure up images of seemingly random objects, animals, or people. What appears to be random is actually your subconscious mind revealing messages to you, and if you learn to interpret these messages you can reap the rewards of listening to your internal guidance system. You can also speak back to your subconscious using symbolic gestures, colors, and items to create closures in areas of your life where you feel emotional deficits. In this way, you can work with the crystals as representations not of attributes that you lack but of attributes that are already within you that are being called forward. You can view the chakras as a designated map of your emotional body to work through step by step, rather than feeling you need to see these various colors believed in (and sometimes seen and felt) by others.

“ THE MOST IMPORTANT
FACTOR IS HOW SOMETHING
MAKES YOU *FEEL.* ”

For all the practices provided in this book, you may add symbols that are meaningful to you in relation to the exercise. Remember that although there is a collective understanding and acceptance of the meaning of certain symbols, other things will mean something different depending on the person. A great example of this comes from Will Phillips's *Every Dreamer's Handbook*: A dog may represent loyalty and friendship to someone else, but if you were bitten by your childhood dog when you were young, it may represent danger and betrayal to you.

When choosing items to represent the energy that you will be calling forth or focusing on, the most important factor is how something makes you *feel.* For example, let's say you are choosing a piece of art to hang above your bed. One of your choices is an expensive Jackson Pollock print, with wild splatters of multiple colors spinning across the canvas, and it makes you feel on edge. The other one, by an unknown artist, is a clean abstract with peaceful tones, and it makes you feel serene. Although you may think that it'd be more impressive to have a painting by the famous Jackson Pollock in your bedroom, you might choose the more tranquil painting to satisfy your desire to present a more tranquil environment—the one that invokes the feelings you want to create.

There are symbols in our world that have a universal truth, but it is useful and fun to create your own symbolic dictionary based on your personal associations with these symbols. Things that stick out to you from childhood hold keys to understanding your subconscious motives and perhaps even your soul's path. They include the colors you asked your parents to paint your room, your favorite toy, the statue at your grandmother's house, or your favorite childhood movie. Deconstructing the meaning of the objects that stand out in your mind and figuring out the symbolic significance of what they mean to you will help you unlock the way your subconscious is working with you. You can then work with it by meticulously picking out representations from your personal symbol dictionary. This creates a more powerful and intimate experience and one that you may build throughout your life.

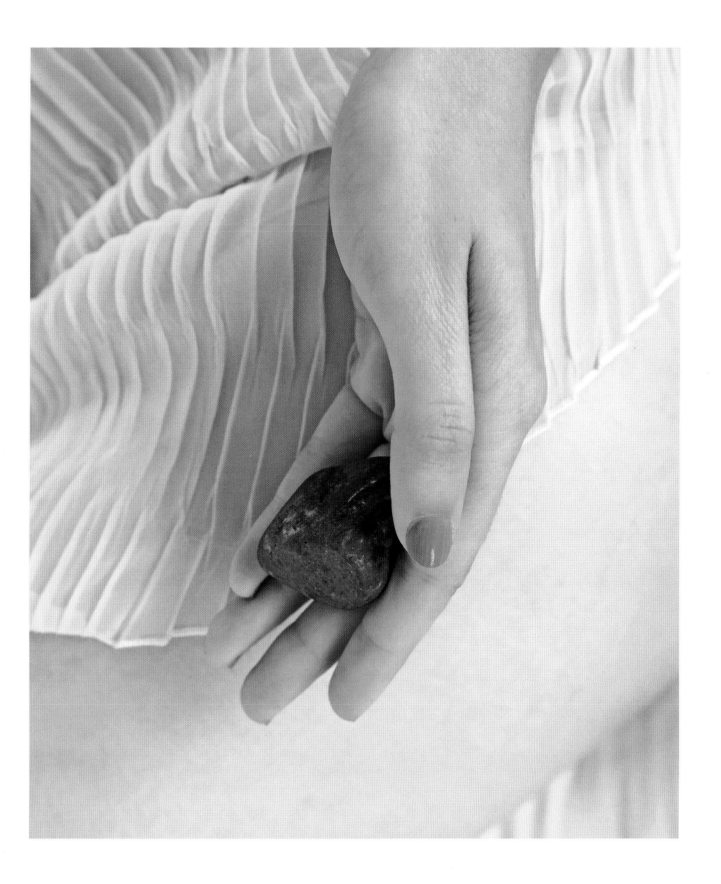

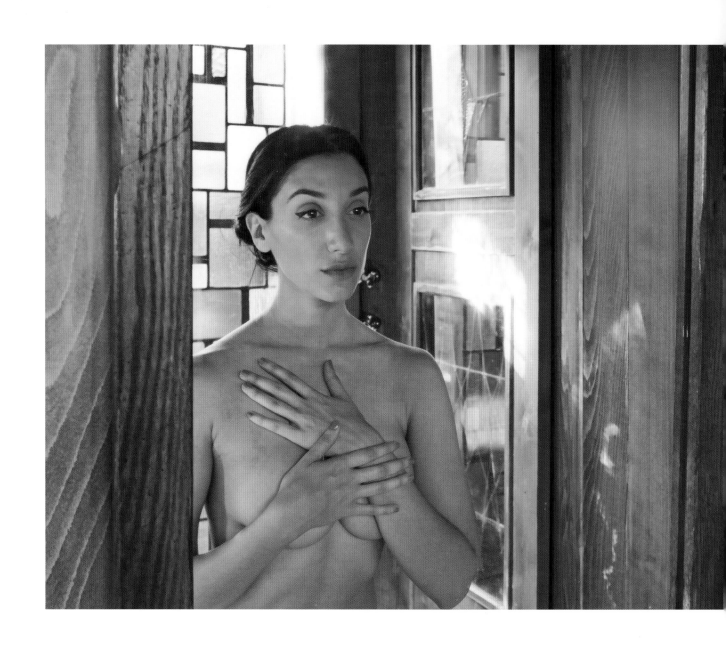

SELF-LOVE IS CARING ABOUT YOURSELF,
BEYOND WHAT YOU SEE IN THE MIRROR.

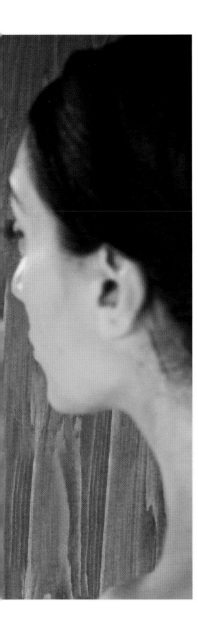

What Self-Love Is Not

"Love yourself." It's the anthem of a new generation, echoing throughout magazines, YouTube videos, and blogs. It's great that so much emphasis is being given to positive self-image. We're seeing more diverse body types, ethnicities, and differently-abled people being represented in mainstream media every day. Although ideas of conventional beauty are being challenged, these positive changes would be even better if we understood what *love* truly is.

What does "self-love" really look like? Self-love is knowing that you are human and that your thoughts and feelings are normal. Real self-love is not identifying yourself with your moods, history, or thoughts. Self-love isn't always beautiful. Self-love is looking at yourself in the mirror with a pimply face and not letting it get to you. Self-love is *not* calling that person that you know deep down is going to distract or hurt you. Self-love is wanting to have that drink to numb the pain but making yourself some tea instead.

Self-love is doing what is best for you—even when you think you're undeserving. Real self-love is simply love. It resides inside you at all times. You are what real self-love is. It looks like you.

There will always be days when looking in the mirror causes discomfort. This is natural. The important thing is to not allow self-destructive thoughts to overwhelm you but to interrupt them with an act of self-love, like listening to music, writing down your thoughts, or drinking some water.

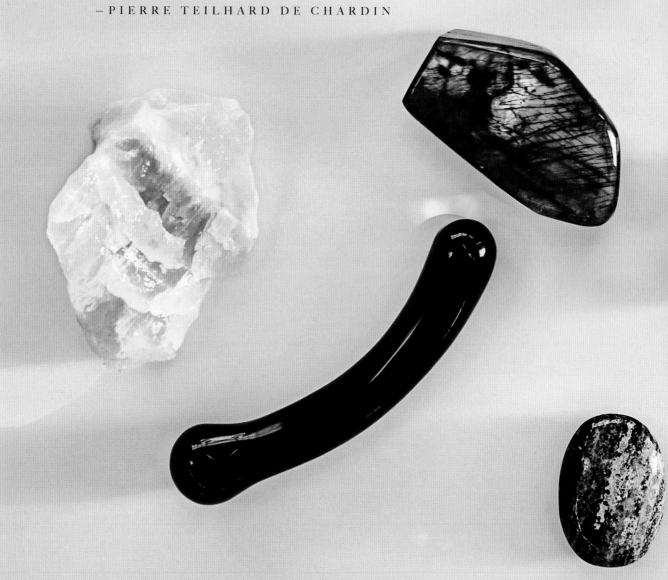

"We are not human beings having a
spiritual experience. We are spiritual beings having
a human experience."

— PIERRE TEILHARD DE CHARDIN

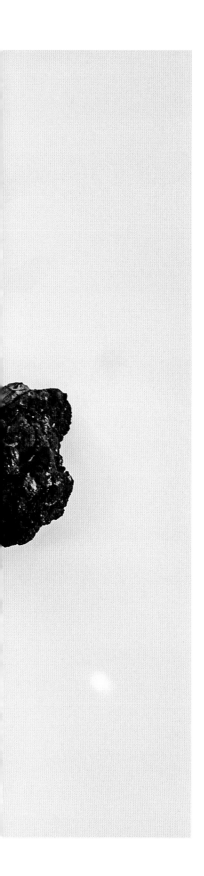

Drink in Love

You can infuse water with rose quartz energy by placing some rose quartz in a container with water overnight. Remove the crystal before drinking the water and receive that loving hydration.

The difference here is that in true love for yourself, you allow yourself to feel a range of complex emotions. It's about understanding that moments of insecurity are just *moments*. It's about becoming self-aware enough that you begin to take note of the fact that your moods do not define you and that everything will pass. It's allowing yourself to feel compassion for yourself; that is an act of self-love. If you're feeling sad, try to connect to that feeling. Love your lonely, love your sadness—love them because they are part of you. Think of yourself as a spirit experiencing a human moment, and recognize it as special. This will create true acceptance of your feelings.

Do not attach yourself to the thoughts that arise when you're feeling down or view them as the absolute truth. Instead, see them as ships passing by. Acknowledge their existence and allow them to move on. Give yourself permission to feel whatever comes up. It is the culmination of these moments—the good and the bad—that make up our rich human experience.

In this way, self-love is more like "self-awareness." It is being present for yourself when you're experiencing low emotions and not making it worse by criticizing yourself for it. Instead, it is becoming a "parent" (or "apparent") to yourself, one who loves you unconditionally. It is seeing your emotions as important to developing who you are. And it is proceeding with care by making yourself comfortable as you experience the momentary feeling.

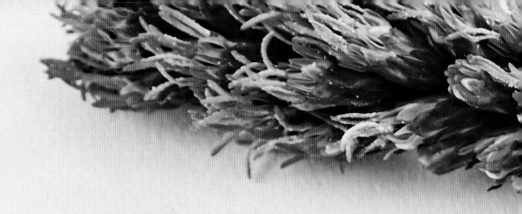

Harmony of Emotions:
FEEL IT ALL, IT'S ALL LOVE

My mother taught me about love when I was learning my opposites. She would say a word like "light" or "dark," and I would say its opposite. One day she said "love," to which I said, "hate." "No, Vanessa," she told me. "The opposite of love is *apathy*, which means the absence of emotion. Love is the culmination of all emotion."

Love is regarded as the highest vibrational emotion there is, because it is the harmony of all emotions. Just as we have to mature our perception of what magic is, we have to mature our perception of love. We assume that love is something that comes naturally. That love is just there, something we experience or we don't. But love can be also seen as an art form that we can study and practice, just as a musician learns her instrument. And just as any musician might tell you about music, in love, there is always more to learn.

Being in a state of love requires finding harmony with your emotions and learning to work with what you're feeling instead of opposing your natural instincts. Our emotions work as intermediaries to our higher intuition, links between the physical world and subtle energies. When we learn to work with—rather than against—our emotions, we can understand the values and lessons that they bring. This is important when engaging in self-development work. You cannot *rid* yourself of emotions you deem "negative," but you can help yourself by allowing them to flow through you and honoring what they are trying to communicate.

Suppressing emotions creates tension and uses energy—energy that could otherwise be used for positive change. When we suppress emotions, we try to place restrictions on what we feel. Repressing an emotion goes even further; we are trying to control the outcome of how we feel. But unprocessed emotions can hurt you. According to Synthia Andrews in her book *The Path of Emotions*, these sentiments may lead to physical symptoms like shaking or trembling, attitudes or beliefs that could hold you back, or even outbursts and overreactions. Because crystals are amplifiers and facilitate movement of energy, they support the fulfillment of suppressed and repressed emotions so they can be acknowledged and flow through the body.

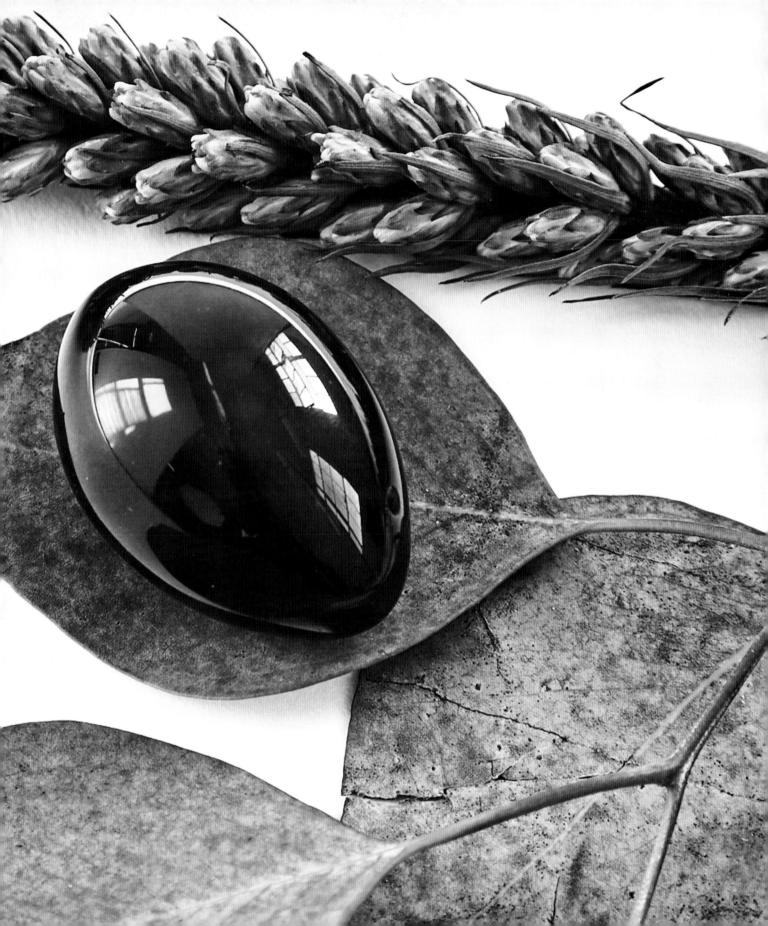

"MAKING PEACE WITH YOUR EMOTIONS IS AS SIMPLE AS PLACING VALUE ON THEM WHEN THEY ARISE."

Unfortunately, too many of us have repressed or suppressed emotions regarding our sexuality or sexual experiences. We are not necessarily given tools to process the emotions that arise when we first enter the world of sexual expression, therefore even non-violent acts of sexuality can become traumatic.

For example, when I experienced intercourse for the first time, I wasn't aware that it was going to happen. Without my consent, it could be considered sexual assault, but because it wasn't inherently "violent," I didn't see it that way. After working with my obsidian Chakrub, I learned that entering into someone without consent is itself an act of violence. I discovered that I had been repressing my anger and sadness for years. I'd become completely numb in my vagina, since this area was the source of my pain. After acknowledging my repressed emotions, I allowed them to be integrated into my life. This led me to understand that I had real anger issues, meaning that I never got angry. Any time I felt angry, I would turn it back on myself. After a few years of working with crystals, and learning how to let anger flow through me, I was finally able to confront my ex-boyfriend, letting him know how angry I was at him, how his actions had affected me, and that I was finally able to understand that what he did to me was wrong. Somewhat surprisingly, his response was, "I know, and I am so sorry." This felt like a victory for me. I was able to forgive him and to allow my anger to flow. We don't always have the opportunity to confront the people who hurt us, but we always have the opportunity to work within our own hearts and to offer ourselves the comfort we need to process our experiences.

Making peace with the full spectrum of our emotions means that we don't limit the flow of energy. Living in harmony with what we feel gives us a greater understanding of how we are communicating with the subtle energy at work within and around us at any given moment. Making peace with your emotions is as simple as placing value on them when they arise and discerning what messages they are bringing. From there, we can let them flow and proceed to act from a place of self-love.

Instant *and* Lasting Gratification

We all know how to soothe ourselves, in moments of low emotions, with quick solutions that do not solve the underlying issue. Mindless eating, consuming alcohol, impulse shopping—and even indulging in sexual acts—may create pleasure in the moment, but they are only temporary fixes. There are times when it's valuable to create pleasure just for pleasure's sake. But when we use a substance or act to dissociate from ourselves or our problems, it's more valuable to get to the root of the issue.

Throughout this book, we will find ways to create lasting gratification by embracing a range of practices for attaining self-pleasure. Introducing crystals and their practical applications for healing to the process is how we make self-pleasure transformative and lasting. The practices in this book incorporate immediate pleasure using physical touch or relaxation techniques alongside methods that alter the vibrational factors of the issues at hand with crystals.

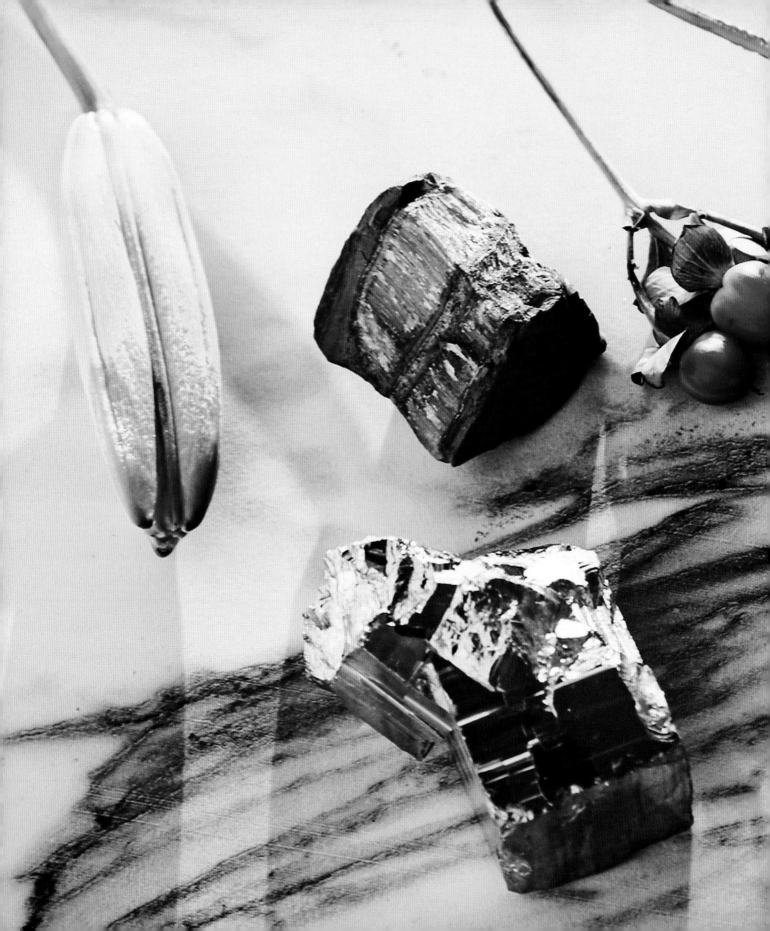

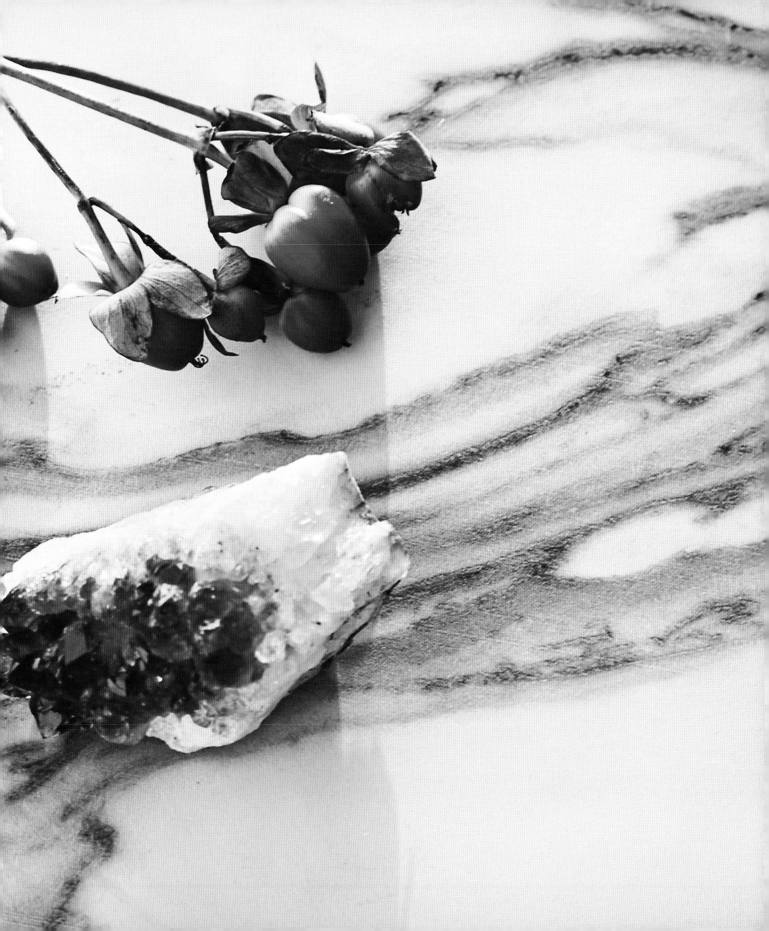

Tools and Techniques for Building Energy

Although we don't necessarily *need* anything outside of ourselves to build energy, as humans we've always created tools to help us. Crystals help move stagnant or low vibrational energy within us by clearing our internal environment, while they keep us grounded by being earth elements. Combining crystals with breathing and other techniques will enhance your experience and offer an anchor of support and added metaphysical benefits.

Crystals are energy amplifiers. When you open yourself to sensing the subtle vibration of crystals, you can sensitize yourself to feeling pleasure more intensely, if you so choose. As we are bombarded with constant stimuli, we need to be reminded of the value of slowing down and being mindful of what we are doing—placing importance on how we expend our energy. If you want to feel crystal energy, the energy of your partner, or the energy of yourself, you have to slow down and practice being open. Any resistance you feel is a signal that you have a great need for this kind of practice.

Being able to meditate, be mindful, and tune in to subtle energy takes muscle. This muscle gets stronger the more you use it.

Many sexuality coaches, if not all, use various powerful tools to help encourage energy movement, including breath, physical movement, visualization, and sound. These are natural partners for crystals. Because crystals amplify and facilitate the movement of energy, we can focus our intention, our sexual energy, by incorporating these tools.

Becoming Whole

Crystals can help us reach different facets of our sexual personalities. Doing so can help us recognize things about ourselves that we may not be aware of. Working through the chakra map, we'll identify areas of ourselves that can be tapped into for more fulfilling sex, relationships, and life.

We are infinite beings capable of accessing a countless range of emotions and traits. We each encompass every characteristic, and discovering this can lead to total self-empowerment.

Crystals serve as physical manifestations of the energetic properties we want to draw forth from ourselves. As amplifiers, crystals will strengthen dormant energy within us, but they do not discriminate.

Aspects of ourselves that we deem "negative" are only negative because of our judgments of them. As long as we are not putting ourselves or anyone else in harm, we can transform our "negative" qualities into something positive through compassion for ourselves.

Obsidian is a crystal that is feared by some, who say it has "bad" energy. This is because obsidian brings to the surface repressed parts of ourselves that we have subconsciously shunned. Early mirrors were made from obsidian. This black, volcanic glass reflects back to you what you may be ignoring about yourself and, at first, you may not like it. It is not actually the crystal that has "bad" energy, but it can show you things that you *think* are bad.

Part of my work with black crystals such as obsidian and onyx exposed an interest in sexual expressions such as masochism, bondage, and other fetishes. I had to learn to remove my judgment of these sexual expressions and understand that true self-love comes from accepting your "shadow self," which Carl Jung describes as the dark side of your personality.

This led me to create a line of Chakrubs called "The Shadow Line," which is made from obsidian crystal but with more fetish-inspired designs. Regarding these darker desires as valuable expressions of the self takes introspection and requires a state of non-judgment. Once we learn to accept these parts of ourselves, we increase our ability to feel compassion for others.

Removing the need to identify with specific qualities, or being able to identify, even a little bit, with all the qualities, creates a view of yourself that is dynamic and infinite.

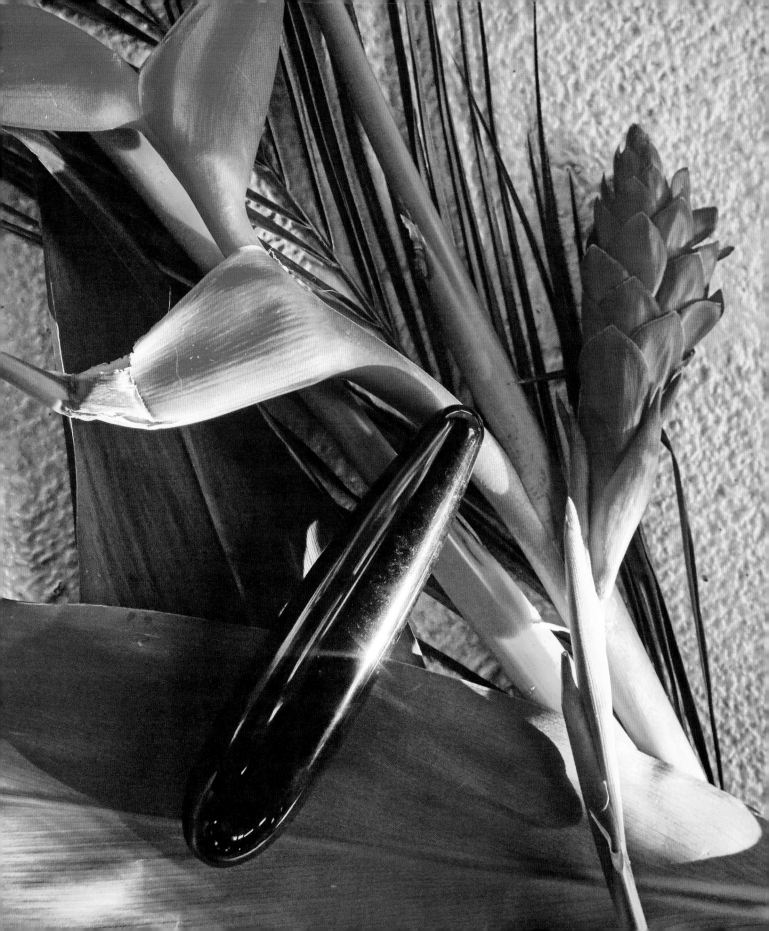

"'This is why alchemy exists,' the boy said. 'So that everyone will search for his treasure, find it, and then want to be better than he was in his former life.'"

— PAULO COELHO, *The Alchemist*

OBSIDIAN CAN HELP
YOU ACKNOWLEDGE AND
CONFRONT REPRESSED
(SOMETIMES DARK)
MEMORIES OR FEELINGS.

Acceptance and Transformation

How can we both accept who we are and at the same time wish to improve ourselves? It seems contradictory. The distinction of *why* we decide to make a change in our lives is an important aspect of self-development. We must hold two truths within our hearts when putting ourselves on this path of improvement: You are perfect, and you are a work in progress.

In order for change to occur, one must acknowledge all parts of the self. You don't need to like everything about who you are—just don't neglect any part of who you are. Every facet of your personality is like a character in a play. Some characters are clumsy, manipulative, or abrasive, but each character serves a purpose in telling the story, making the experience of viewing the play rich with depth and range. Allow all your characters to play their part and get to understand the significance of their roles.

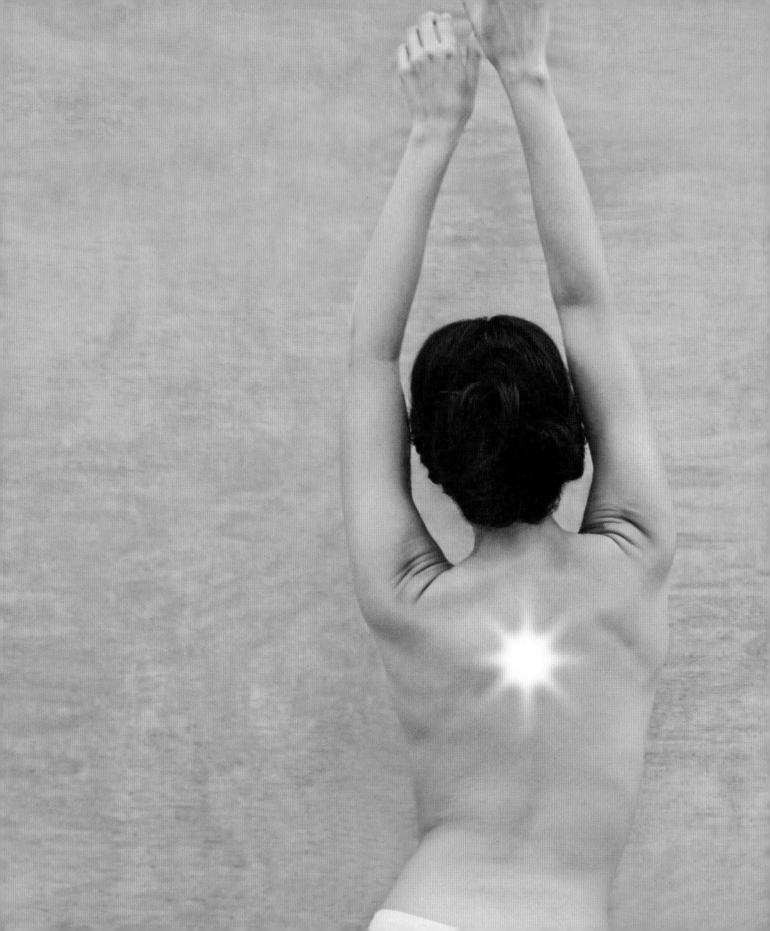

2 | THE CHAKRAS

Our current understanding of the chakra system is drawn from the Hindu tradition that was popularized by the Theosophists at the beginning of the twentieth century. Many of its core teachings originated in the Upanishad texts, dating back to between 800 and 400 BCE.

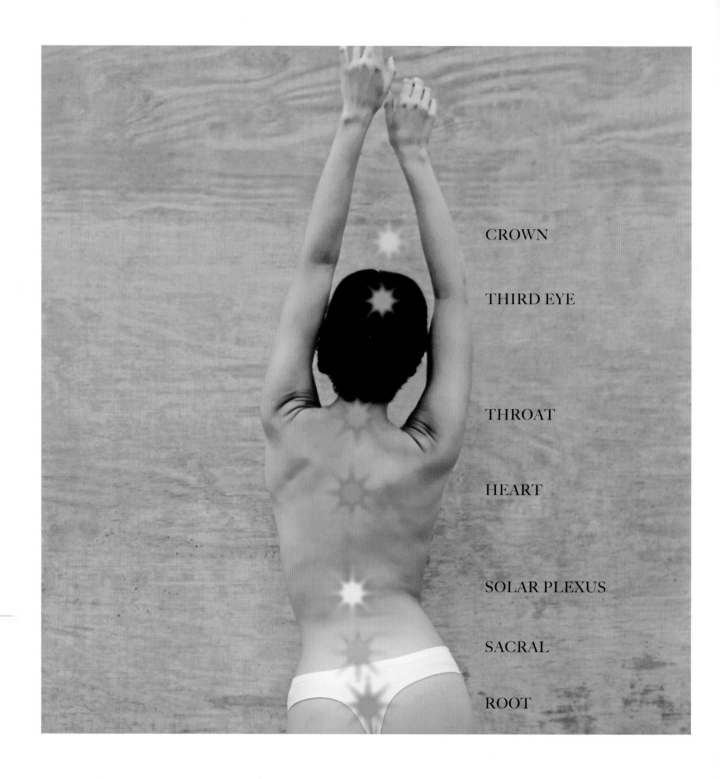

CROWN

THIRD EYE

THROAT

HEART

SOLAR PLEXUS

SACRAL

ROOT

Word Origin: Chakra

The term *chakra* derives from a word in the ancient East Indian language Sanskrit meaning "spinning wheel," as a healthy chakra functions by spinning easily.

Chakras are points of energy in our bodies that carry out specific functions for physical, psychological, and spiritual purposes. Chakras can interact with different kinds of energy, some of which we can detect and see, some of which we cannot. They are described as vortexes, as portals of consciousness, each one a key to unlocking depth in awareness. There are thousands of these points in our bodies, but in this book we will focus on the Western understanding of the seven that make up the chakra system.

Properties of the Chakras

Many people can sense their chakra system. Some can feel their chakras spinning or pulsing, or hear them as tones. Some see them as colors; the ancients used their intuition to sense the colors of the chakras, and the seven main chakras correspond to the colors of the rainbow. At the base of the spine, the root chakra is considered red, and up at the top of the head, the crown chakra is violet. Every color vibrates at a different speed or frequency; for example, red has a lower frequency and violet has a higher frequency.

In this system, the lower chakras have to do with earthly and physical needs, whereas the higher ones operate with the spiritual planes. The chakras are also linked to different notes on the musical scale. Though there are many variations, I like to think of the root as "C," going up the C major scale as you go up the chakras. Every tone of the musical scale also vibrates at a different frequency; the lower the tone, the slower the vibration. The chakras correlate to the elements, personality archetypes, senses, and the endocrine and nervous systems.

Acknowledging your sensitivity to a range of subtle energies is a way to find clarity when issues arise. Each situation you encounter is an opportunity to access your innermost wisdom and find guidance to learn a positive lesson. It's as if you will understand the language of your spirit.

In *The Complete Book of Chakra Healing*, Cyndi Dale explains that there are three main functions of the chakras: physical processing, psychological processing, and spiritual processing. Chakras in the seven-chakra system have a location in the body and are each attached to a nerve plexus and/or endocrine gland. The nerve plexuses and endocrine glands they are associated with are how we detect what energy center needs attention based on physical ailments. Emotions act as a conduit for our physical realm and spiritual realm, because they are energy we can feel. Our emotional well-being is constructed through our beliefs, and each chakra aides in those

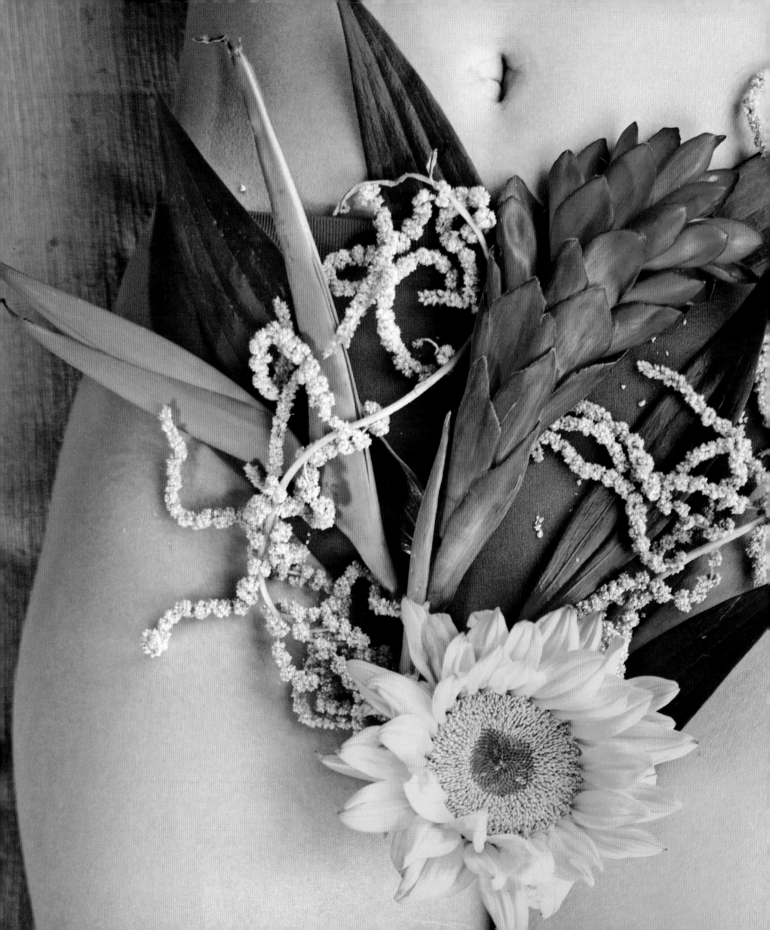

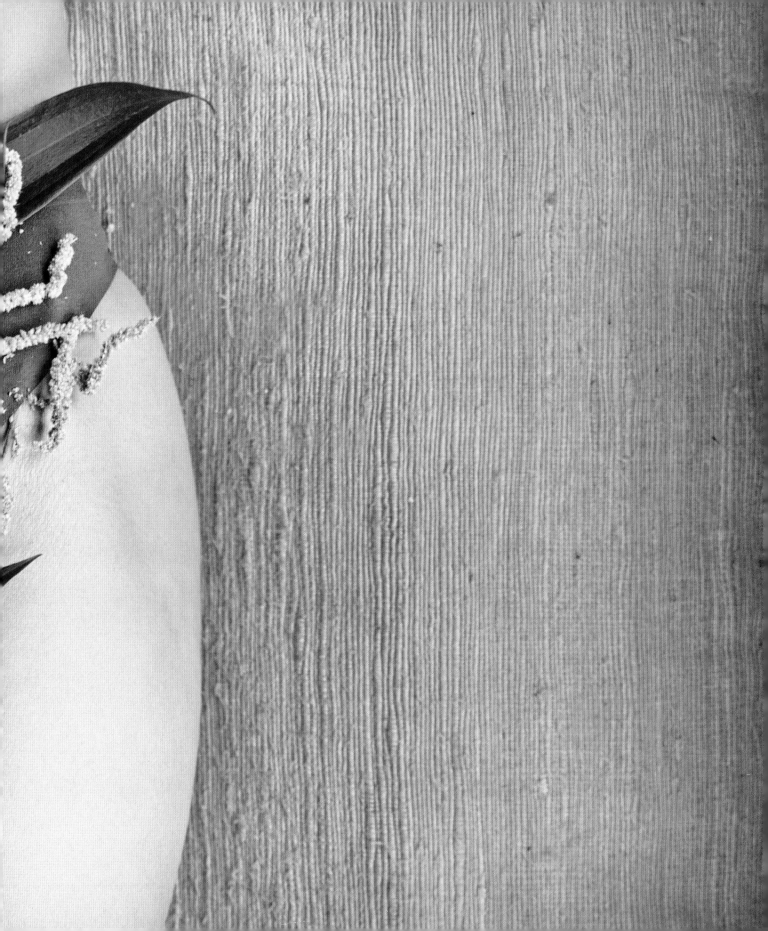

psychological constructs. The spiritual aspect of the chakras adds a layer of awareness of ourselves as we evolve our sense of self. Psychic abilities such as clairvoyance, clairaudience, clairsentience, and claircognizance are also governed through these centers. When working up the ladder of chakras starting at the base, you also work up the ladder of enlightenment, which is a sense of universal understanding that cannot be put into words.

Chakras respond to stimuli, and they can be nurtured through our attention to them. Ideally, they are dynamic, opening and closing based on our needs. They are record keepers and transformers of our energy, meaning they have memory of our emotional responses to events. They can also transform physical energy into subtle energy and back.

Chakras and Sex

Being aware of the chakra system helps open the door to experience it yourself. For years, I had been drawn to and studied this system. I love how it neatly organizes a wide range of what is necessary to focus on for self-development: From primal instincts to emotional health and spiritual attunement, this system covers it all. Because I was open to this system, I achieved a better understanding when my friend Michelle performed Reiki on me. Reiki is a type of energy healing with which certified practitioners channel universal energy to an individual to help create flow in the body. It uses the chakra system. When Michelle performed Reiki, without touching me, her hands moved over my chest and caused me to suddenly burst out in tears from the intensity I felt in my heart. This was unexpected, uncontrollable, and wonderful. A year later, at a tantra workshop given by Barbara Carrellas, I learned a similar technique for moving energy through the chakra system, but this time it was of a sexual nature. Through moaning, breathing, and focused attention, I learned to move my sexual energy up my chakra system, and again, when it reached my heart, I began to cry. This is called an energy orgasm or *breathgasm*, as Carrellas explains in her book, *Urban Tantra*.

I don't really know what everyone else's experience was during that workshop, but for me it was profound. Trust me, I didn't want to be crying profusely while surrounded by people trying to learn to achieve touchless orgasm. But it didn't matter. I experienced a release of energy in my heart that made me cry. We teach what it is we need to learn the most; self-love, what I am most noted for teaching, is my hardest lesson. My heart carries so much energy that it becomes vital for me to do the chakra healing exercises in this book regularly. Even if you don't initially sense your chakras, simply learning about them allows you to open your ability to really tune in to them, which could help you invigorate them. When I experienced my heartgasm, it felt exactly like what it sounds like—an orgasm in my heart. Conjuring your sexual energy and visualizing it in the different points of your body is the easiest way to sense your chakras, which can also help you heal them. (See page 179 for a version of the energy orgasm that was originally made popular by Annie Sprinkles and Barbara Carrellas. It has been modified to involve the use of crystals, further enhancing its effects.)

Our base and sacral chakras are the most commonly discussed chakras when it comes to sexuality, but each chakra lends its particular energy force to the overall sensual experience. Working with the chakra system helps focus our attention on multifaceted areas of life, including sexuality.

"EACH CHAKRA LENDS ITS PARTICULAR ENERGY FORCE TO THE OVERALL SENSUAL EXPERIENCE."

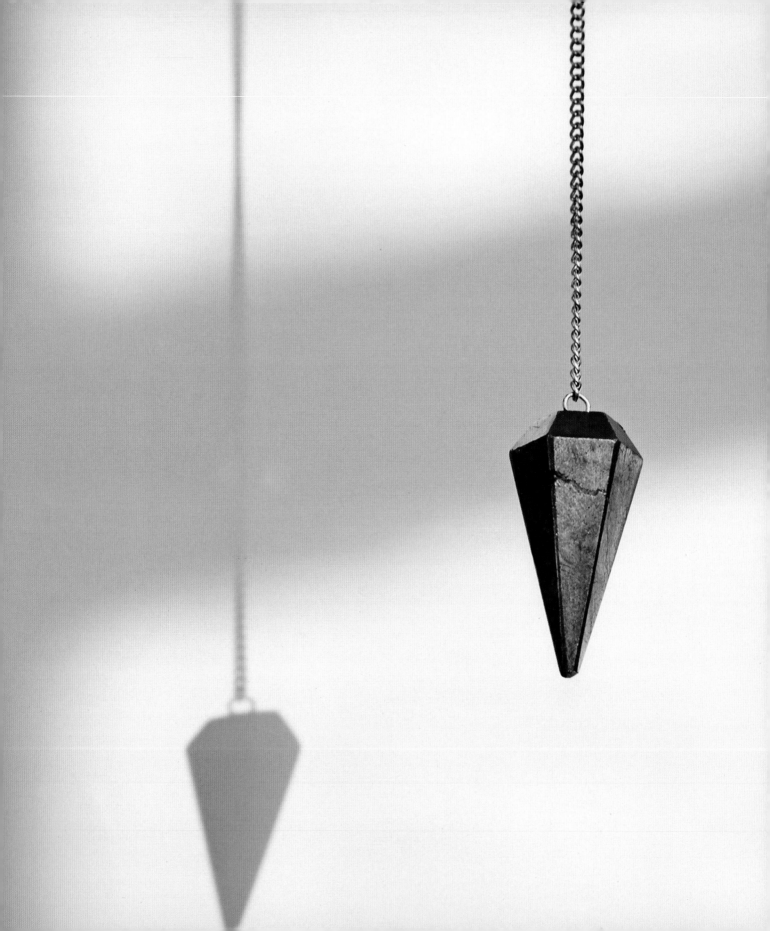

A PENDULUM CAN BE USED TO
IDENTIFY BLOCKED CHAKRAS.
HOLD A PENDULUM OVER A
PARTICULAR CHAKRA FOR A
MOMENT. IF IT SWINGS SIDE
TO SIDE, IT IS BLOCKED. IF IT
CIRCULATES, IT IS OPEN.

Blocked Chakras

Because chakras are dynamic, we can experience a chakra feeling very open in one situation but closed in another. For example, we may find that our heart chakra is open when we are around long-time friends and family and feel we can easily give and receive love, but then it may close when we find ourselves on a first date with a potential lover. One way to balance a chakra that we want to remain more open in certain situations is to recognize when we feel open in those situations and call upon that feeling that needs more support. The practices in this book will help nourish each chakra and raise awareness of what it *feels* like to have a healthy and balanced chakra system.

When we talk about chakras being open, it means that they are functioning properly. When a chakra is closed, it doesn't mean it's completely shut but rather that there are blocks or inhibitions due to or issues stored within it.

When a chakra is blocked, it means that there is subtle energy inhibiting the full range of its function. This could be trapped emotions from not understanding how to process something, it could be an imbedded mental idea, or it could even be another person's energy. When you are being intimate with someone, especially in moments of deep pleasure, channels between the two of you open wide and may carry debris. You can release these blockages by clearing and cleansing the chakras.

Balancing and aligning the chakras means both making sure each individual chakra is in alignment (the front and back side are equal), and that each one is operating with the others at an optimum level.

The root cause of ailments, be they physical, emotional, or spiritual, is energy, because everything is energy. We must seek out medical treatments and professional assistance when appropriate and look to practices that support our energy systems as complementary—not in lieu of traditional—treatment. By acknowledging the reality of energy as part of our existence, we further support ourselves in the pursuit of complete well-being.

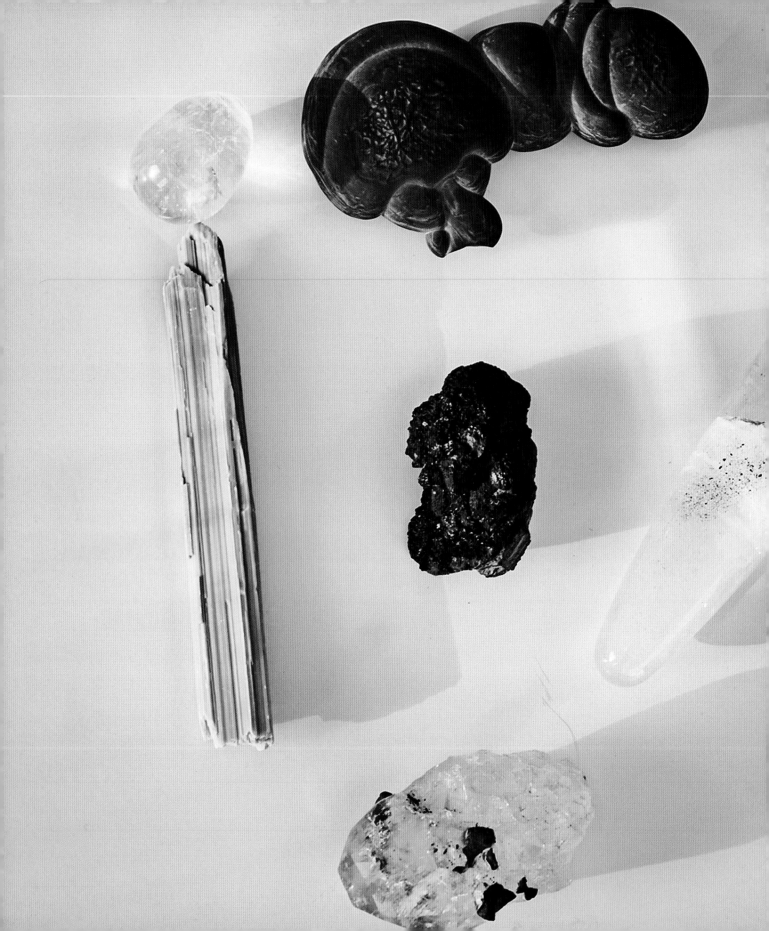

3 | THE WORLD OF CRYSTALS

As far back as we have recorded human history, crystals have had a role to play. For example, the word *amethyst* comes from an ancient Greek word meaning "not intoxicating." The ancient Greeks would carry around an amethyst on a night of drinking because they believed it would help them keep a sober mind. Today, we recognize amethyst for its calming energy, and it is useful for those needing support when releasing an addiction or habit.

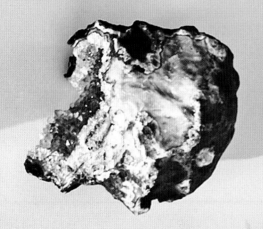

The Hindu link between crystals and subtle energy dates all the way back to the *Rig Veda*, an ancient Indian collection of Vedic Sanskrit hymns that recommends using seven gems to capture the sun's rays. In the Puranas, a collection of religious and mythical Hindu literature, crystals were associated with areas of the body, the nine planets of our solar system, and fixtures in Vedic astrology.

Crystal Uses Throughout History

Talismans and amulets date back to the beginning of humankind; Baltic amber amulets that were discovered in Britain date back to 30,000 years ago. People all over the world have found practical uses for and spiritual connections with crystals ever since.

Ancient Egyptians used lapis lazuli, turquoise, carnelian, emerald, and clear quartz in their jewelry and for grave amulets. But they used stones primarily for protection and health. Chrysolite (later translated as both topaz and peridot), for example, was used to combat night terrors and to purge evil spirits.

Egyptians also used crystals cosmetically. Galena (lead ore) was ground to a powder and used as the eye shadow known as kohl. Malachite was used in a similar manner. Green-toned crystals, such as fluorite, amazonite, and emerald, were used to signify the heart of the deceased in burials. Green stones were used in a similar way at a later period in ancient Mexico.

The ancient Greeks believed crystals to have numerous benefits. Many of the crystal-related names we use today are of Greek origin. In fact, the word *crystal* itself comes from the Greek word for ice, as it was believed that clear quartz was water that had frozen so deeply that it would always remain solid. *Hematite* comes from the word for blood, because of the red coloration produced when it oxidizes. Hematite is an iron ore; the ancient Greeks associated iron with Ares, the god of war. Greek soldiers would rub hematite over their bodies before battle, purportedly to make themselves invulnerable. Greek sailors also wore a variety of amulets to keep them safe at sea.

Jade was incredibly valuable in ancient China. Chimes were made from jade, and some ancient Chinese emperors were buried in jade armor. Burials with jade masks also occurred around the same period in Mexico. Jade was recognized as a kidney healing stone in both China and South America.

Two hundred fifty years ago, the Maoris of New Zealand wore jade pendants representing ancestor spirits, which were passed down many generations through the male line. The tradition of green stones being lucky continues in parts of New Zealand to present day.

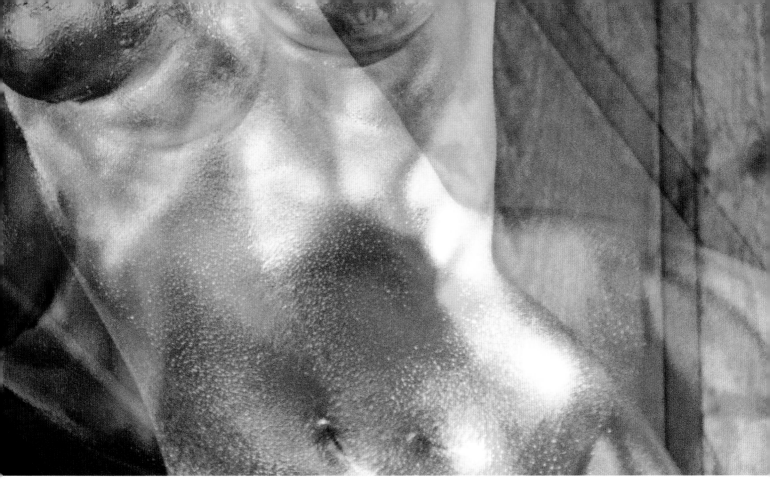

How Crystals Work to Facilitate Energy Movement

Our world is constantly in motion and in communication with itself. Everything in it—from thoughts to colors to furniture—resonates at a vibrational frequency. Frequency is, basically, the speed that molecules rotate around each other. This causes an energetic wave, or vibration. Our vibrational field works in harmony with all other beings, and it is our responsibility to maintain it for collective health and wellness.

Crystals are defined by their incredibly organized internal structures, which are made up of repeating arrangements of atoms known as crystal lattices. These lattices influence what the crystal looks like and categorize them as the most stable state of matter.

When we share a space with a crystal, our energy bodies become more like that of the crystal, rather than the other way around. They superimpose harmonizing patterns of energy currents into the body's energy field, or aura.

There are three categories of rock: igneous, sedimentary, and metamorphic. They include all crystals.

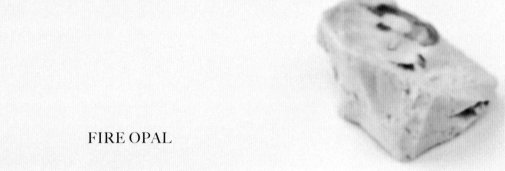

FIRE OPAL

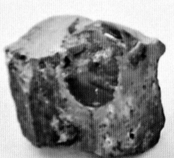

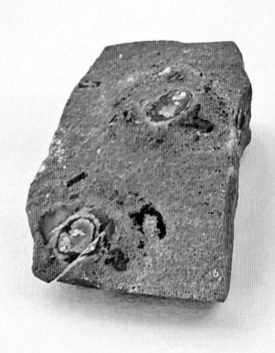

Igneous

Igneous rock is formed when intense pressure forces liquid magma or lava to the surface, where it eventually solidifies into rock. Over time, interlocking gemstones and crystals begin to grow within these rocks. Rock that solidifies underneath the surface is called intrusive; it cools slowly and has coarse mineral grains visible to the naked eye. Rock that hardens above the surface is called extrusive; it cools more quickly and its appearance is smooth, crystalline, and fine-grained. Cooling time, mineralogy, chemical composition, texture, and geometry all affect how igneous rocks are classified.

E X A M P L E S : fire opal, obsidian

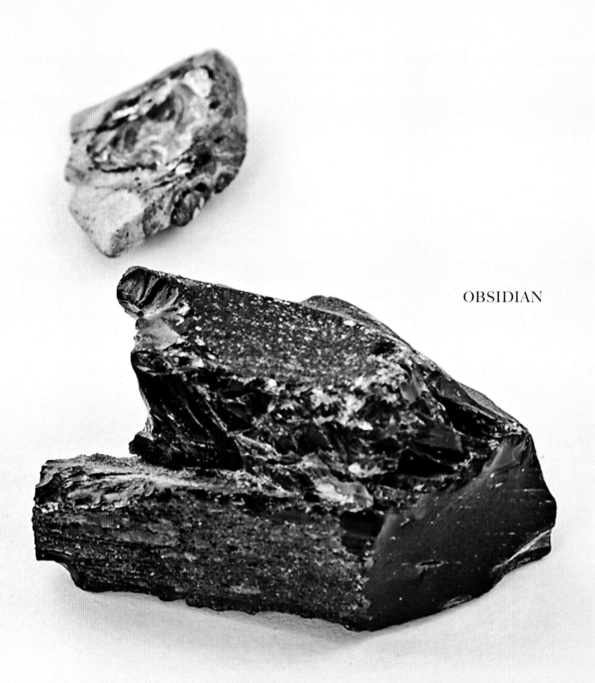

OBSIDIAN

SAPPHIRE

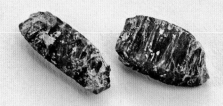

QUARTZ

RUBY

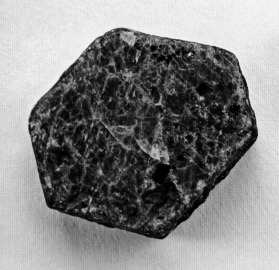

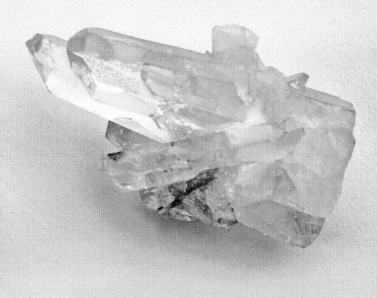

Sedimentary

Sedimentary rocks are formed by the accumulation of mineral particles on the Earth's surface as a result of weather and erosion. Over time, layers of fragments, along with mud and other organic and inorganic elements, are compacted into hard rock. Sedimentary rock covers three-quarters of the Earth's surface, but represents only 8 percent of the total volume of the planet's crust.

E X A M P L E S : ruby, sapphire, quartz

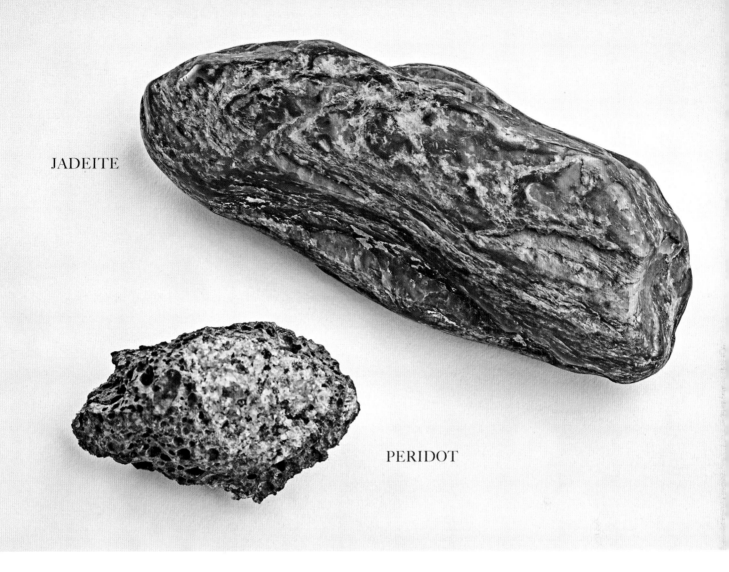

JADEITE

PERIDOT

Metamorphic

Metamorphic rocks are made by recrystallization, which is caused by intense pressure and high temperatures, transforming the composition of a rock deep within the Earth's crust, or through direct contact with hot magma.

E X A M P L E S : jadeite, peridot

Crystals' power comes from how they were created, and the oscillations of their internal structures creating vibrational frequencies. The Earth's crust is composed of magma, liquid rock, that gets pushed up to the surface—by means of volcanic eruption, for example. This process may include intense heating and cooling. While a rock is going on its journey, it may pick up other minerals, which dictates what type of crystal it will become.

When a crystal grows, it develops lattices with gaps in the structure, extra atoms, or atoms of slightly different sizes. So even though crystals are in a state of equilibrium, this leaves a reservoir of extra electrons with nothing to do. We can give these electrons purpose by putting energy into the crystal. This enables crystals to act as transducers and transform one form of energy into another.

Energy is a property with the ability to do work. It can be transformed into other types of energy, but it cannot be created or destroyed. Think of stones as a source of potential energy that transforms into electrical energy when met with a heat source—such as your skin.

I always find it entertaining to ask people in crystal shops why they believe crystals are used in healing. My most recent encounter gave me insight not only on the crystals but on the young woman with whom I was talking. She told me that the power of crystals comes from the process of their creation. She said that their beauty is derived from the struggle they endure while forming. She was correct; crystals do go through a lot to develop as beautifully as they do. And perhaps that is why they are considered such powerful healers. Do you want to learn how to heal from heartbreak from someone who's never been in a relationship? Or do you want to learn from someone who has been through relationship hell and has wisdom gained from how they triumphed? We all go through struggle, pain, and hardships. We all experience it differently. Sometimes the best way to channel great pain is to help others. Crystals can be seen in this light.

The Symbolism of Crystals

As you deepen your understanding of crystals, you'll find that their symbolism is far from random. Each variety of crystal holds potent metaphorical importance through its metaphysical properties, historic uses, color, shape, and configurations. We can reveal vast meaning through each of these elements.

Turquoise, for example, was sacred to ancient Persian and Native American cultures, and it has been celebrated as a symbol of wisdom and prosperity for centuries. It is known to be a strengthening stone and is used for enhancing the immune system. This is connected to its physicality: It is classified as a phosphate, and phosphates are necessary for the formation of bones and teeth and also used by cells in energy production. Strength and more strength.

Another example: Ancient Egyptians placed quartz on the heads of the dead in their tomb to heal their souls and ensure a safe passageway to the afterlife. Today, quartz is widely regarded as the "master healer" stone and is a fundamental crystal in any energy healer's toolbox.

Our understanding of the metaphysical properties of crystals is also part of collective consciousness. Some of what we know about crystals is channeled information from people who can sense the different benefits each variety offers. One such crystal expert is Judy Hall, who is said to "channel" the benefits of crystals through her abilities as a psychic medium. You can channel information from a crystal and sense its properties before you research it to see if you are in tune to the collective understanding of that crystal. Note that while each type of crystal is ascribed to different meanings, each individual crystal has its own entity and holds its own powers.

The rainbow of colors in which we find crystals is meaningful to the different chakras, the elements (such as earth, water, fire, and air), and color therapy. Color therapy, also known as chromotherapy, is a therapy method that uses color vibrations to heal the body. It's based on how colors themselves vibrate at specific rates, which correlate to various physical embodiments.

There is also an understanding that crystals with a "milkier" appearance embody a feminine and receptive energy, and the clearer crystals have a more masculine energy.

According to philosophies set forth by Plato, everything in nature is built upon five geometrical formations called the platonic solids. When crystals form, they replicate these shapes, the building blocks of nature. When crystals have one or more of these formations, they symbolize the element of those platonic solids.

Crystal Shapes

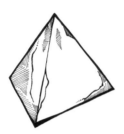

TETRAHEDRON

4 faces; represents element of fire. The fire element represents willpower, inner strength, transformation through action, and passion. Western zodiac representations of fire are Aries, Leo, and Sagittarius. Naturally occurs in Apophyllite crystal.

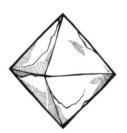

OCTAHEDRON

8 faces; represents the element of air. The air element represents intellect, mental intention, connection to life force, and love. Western zodiac representations of air are Libra, Aquarius, and Gemini. Naturally occurs in diamond crystal.

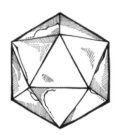

ICOSAHEDRON

20 faces; represents the element of water. The water element represents emotions, being in natural flow. Western Zodiac representations of water are Cancer, Scorpio, and Pisces. Not found in physical nature.

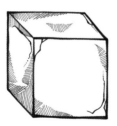

CUBE

6 faces; represents the element of earth. The earth element represents animal instincts, foundation, grounding, and vitality. Western zodiac representation of earth are Capricorn, Taurus, and Virgo. Naturally occurs in pyrite crystal.

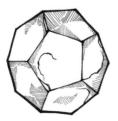

DODECAHEDRON

12 faces; represents the element of spirit. The spirit element represents energy, that which we cannot see. It has no zodiac representations. Naturally occurs in garnet crystal.

Crystal Configurations

Crystals also form in many different configurations. They represent the beneficial energy that the crystals bring forth. Certain stones may have multiple configurations; they don't just need to have one. When choosing crystals to work with, consider the symbolism of their configurations, to add depth to your work with them.

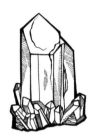

ABUNDANCE STONE

An abundance stone is a single larger piece with a lot of different smaller pieces connected all around it. It's beneficial for taking note of the abundance around you and to wake you up out of a "lacking" energy.

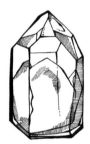

PHANTOM

A phantom is created when one crystal is forming when something happened in the earth and another crystal forms around it. These are beneficial for tapping into your internal guidance system and honoring your intuitive healer.

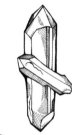

CROSS

A cross is a stone in which two crystals formed crossing each other. It's beneficial for when we feel at a crossroads in life and want added support.

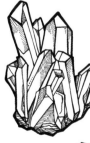

CLUSTER

Multiple points in a naturally occurring crystal cluster remind us that everyone has their own unique point of view, but all people are connected in community. It's great for communication. Clusters may be helpful for people in polyamorous relationships by supporting clear and honest communication.

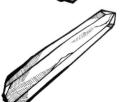

LASER WAND

Naturally formed and usually quartz, laser wands become an extension of the user's intentions and energy. They are excellent tools for breaking up stagnant energy or cutting energetic ties.

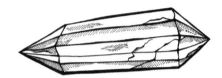

VOGEL WAND

Vogel wands are designed by Marcel Vogel to symbolize the Tree of Life in Kabbalah. Distinguishable by their precise faceting, the female (receptive) end draws in energy, which spirals down the length of the crystal, being amplified every time it hits a facet. This highly amplified energy flows through the male end of the crystal (which is cut at a larger interior angle than the female end), where it is focused into a coherent, laser-like energy.

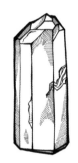

GENERATOR

The faces of a generator crystal are even in size and come together at a point. Generators are considered a strong power source for other crystals, kind of like a battery. They are most often used to charge quartz crystals. Beneficial for meditation and psychic protection.

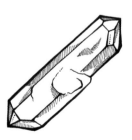

DOUBLE TERMINATED

Double-terminated crystals have a naturally occurring point at both ends. They are helpful for when you want to both receive and give energy in a balanced way. And they're beneficial when you need to nurture a relationship yet also ensure your energy is not being drained. They create circuitry with energy.

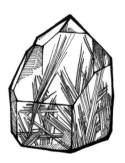

RUTILATED

A rutilated crystal has strands of gold or another mineral within a naturally occurring crystal. It will amplify your intentions and can attract love and stabilize relationships. Rutilated quartz is particularly effective for getting things moving energetically. It can be used for helping slowed chakras return to normal spin and balance. Rutilated quartz is associated with the solar plexus chakra and is sometimes considered a link between the root and crown chakras.

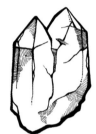

KEY CRYSTAL

A key crystal has a small cavity that was created by another crystal's presence but was later removed. This configuration can be useful when you want to open up to different types of healing modalities (such as crystal or energy healing), or to gain a key insight to a situation.

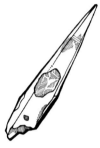

TANTRIC TWIN

A tantric twin crystal has two individual points of the same height, growing together at a base. This type of configuration is beneficial for one-on-one relationships. There are different types of twin configurations, including Gemini Twin, which has two crystal points growing from the same base, but that are clearly different crystal varieties.

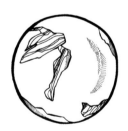

SPHERE

This is a polished, man-made crystal sphere. Because they have no beginning or end, spheres support our intentions in the present moment. They represent completion, fullness, and the realization of all possibilities.

You may also encounter certain crystals that are carved and polished to have a shape that is symbolic of the type of healing it is being called to give. A rose quartz may be carved into a heart—to amplify the intention of feeling love, for example. Animals such as frogs, horses, or birds may be carved to invoke a Native American tradition of animal medicine or spirit guides. Angels, spheres, and skulls are just a few other examples of shapes crystals may be carved in to enhance the energy through their symbolic shapes.

Some crystal shapes have uses that more specifically involve sexuality. You may find one of these particularly helpful for the exercises in this book.

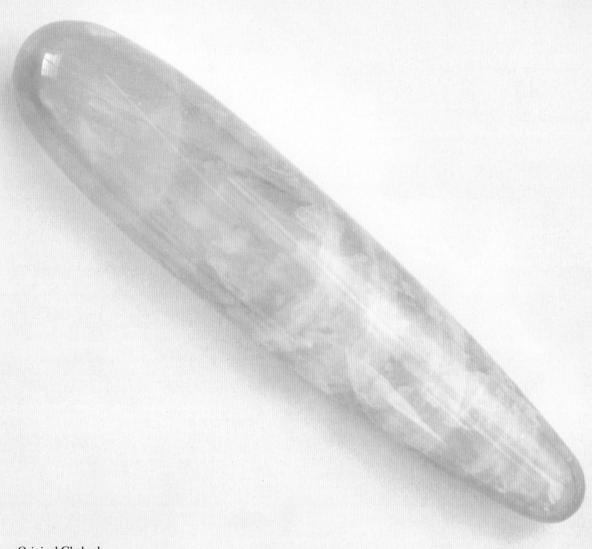

Original Chakrub:

An Original Chakrub is a cylindrical wand that gradually gets larger from one end to the next. Note that it's representative of the sacred space within a vagina, rather than a phallic symbol. Chakrubs are a way for many to experience pleasure without the underlying implication that a penis is required. Chakrubs are created from the "mother stone," a large chunk of crystal that is polished down and shaped to be delivered to the owner, never having been previously owned.

Caution: Chakrubs are created specifically for use as intimate massagers. Crystal "wands" that you may find at new age stores are polished into wand shapes just like the animal or other shapes mentioned previously. These "wands" should not be used internally, not only because they may have been previously owned and thus have another person's energies and may not be hygienic, but because they may be made of stone that isn't recommended for internal use. Certain crystals, such as selenite, should not get wet.

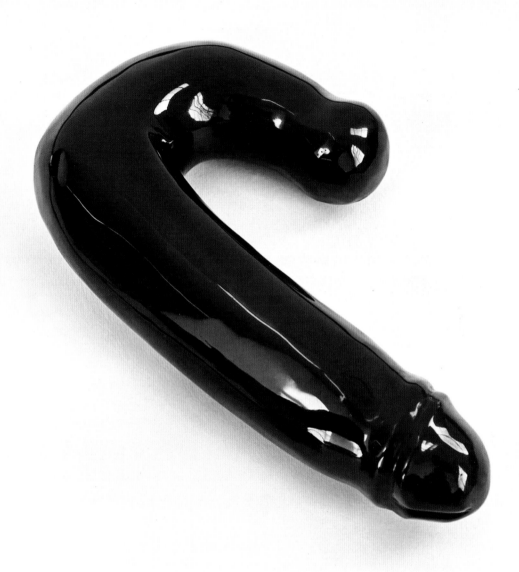

Chakrub Diletto:

This Chakrub is shaped more like a penis. Often when phallic symbols are carved out of crystal, they are seen as a representation of masculine energy. They are also seen as a sign of strength and fertility, and they can be used to heal from sexual trauma or shame. We can work with these stones when we want to provide energy and tap into our masculinity. We all have masculine and feminine energy present in our energy field, regardless of our gender identity. Vulvas and phallic symbols can be used to work with these energies when there is an imbalance.

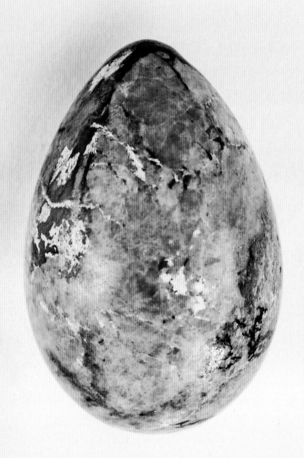

Yoni egg:

Yoni eggs are special crystals carved and polished to resemble an egg. *Yoni* is a Sanskrit word meaning "source," "womb," and "vulva." The yoni egg practice involves inserting the egg into the vagina and engaging the pelvic floor to do exercises with it inside. Some eggs come with a drilled hole in the middle for use with a string, to perform advanced yoni egg practices. Although this practice has gained popularity in the past several years, it is an ancient Chinese practice dating back more than 2,000 years. Traditionally, a jade egg was used for its heavy weight, which was deemed useful for vaginal exercises to help regain control over the vagina after childbirth. It has also been shown to increase blood flow and promote natural lubrication after menopause.

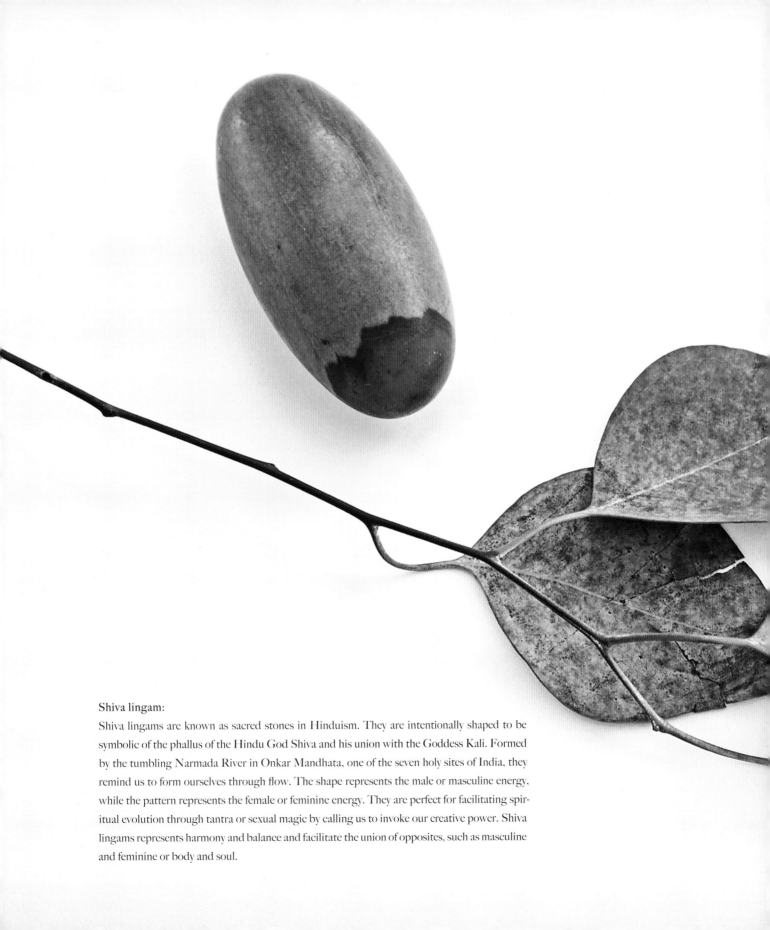

Shiva lingam:

Shiva lingams are known as sacred stones in Hinduism. They are intentionally shaped to be symbolic of the phallus of the Hindu God Shiva and his union with the Goddess Kali. Formed by the tumbling Narmada River in Onkar Mandhata, one of the seven holy sites of India, they remind us to form ourselves through flow. The shape represents the male or masculine energy, while the pattern represents the female or feminine energy. They are perfect for facilitating spiritual evolution through tantra or sexual magic by calling us to invoke our creative power. Shiva lingams represents harmony and balance and facilitate the union of opposites, such as masculine and feminine or body and soul.

"WHEN YOU MAKE THE INITIAL STEPS INTO PURCHASING A NEW CRYSTAL, YOU ARE IN THE PROCESS OF WORKING WITH IT."

While many purveyors of this newly popularized trend say that it is good for "tightening" the vagina, I disregard that wording as I see it as not being body-positive language. When working with a yoni egg, regard it as a tool to *strengthen* yourself not just physically but in terms of the connection you have to your sacred space, womb, vulva, source energy. Being that these are egg-shaped and referred to as "yoni eggs," we are focusing on giving attention to source energy, creative potential, nurturing ideas, and so on. "Birthing" the egg is another way to understand the full range of motion of the vaginal muscles, and to learn how to relax and release tension in the area.

Many different crystal varieties are available to use for this practice. Always do your research when making a purchase and choose a provider who is trusted and knows what crystals are safe for insertion. There are many courses available on the yoni egg practice online and with coaches. Resources are listed in the back of this book.

Choosing Your Crystals

Already, when you make the initial steps into purchasing a new crystal, you are in the process of working with it. Crystals, being that they were formed with the earth, carry a type of consciousness within them that we do not yet fully understand. Many serious crystal healers believe that when you choose a crystal, it has actually already chosen *you*. Once you begin appreciating crystals and working with them, you'll start feeling drawn to them in inexplicable ways. There have been many times in my life that I've been in a new city and I happen to walk into a souvenir shop that has nothing to do with metaphysics, and find my way over to a little hidden section in the shop with some crystals for sale. There have also been times when I've gone to a crystal shop and been struck by the beauty of a crystal, but when I hold it in my hand, I know that it isn't for me. Though this is sometimes disappointing, choosing crystals is all about listening to your intuition. The process of choosing crystals is a great start to honoring your inner wisdom, because you really can't make a mistake.

There are times when I've felt uncertain about crystals that I've acquired, and that becomes a mirror for me to observe the part of myself that sometimes feels insecure about decisions I make. In that way, they were the right crystals to choose.

When making a purchase, it is always a good idea and gracious act to seek out trusted retailers of crystals who are knowledgeable about the origins of the crystals to ensure that they were ethically sourced and mined. Supporting small businesses could also be a factor in the positive energy you create when making a purchase that will carry through to working with your new crystal.

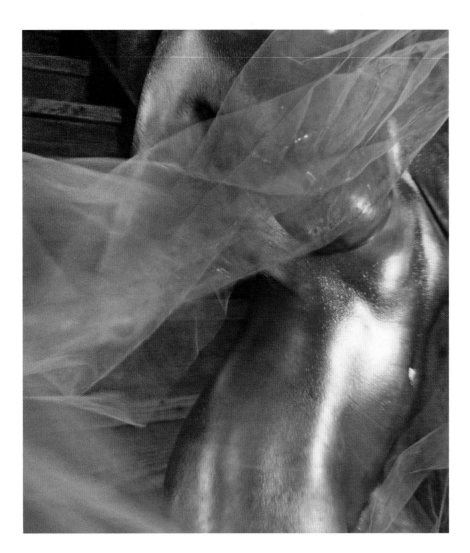

VISUALIZE GOLDEN LIGHT SURROUNDING YOU TO PROTECT
YOURSELF FROM PICKING UP ON OTHER PEOPLE'S ENERGY.

When purchasing your crystals from a physical shop, you have the opportunity to spend time with different ones, tuning in to their energy to feel what's right for you. When I go to metaphysical shops, I can sometimes feel overwhelmed by all the crystals, mystical products, and even the people working there. If you are sensitive, you may find it beneficial to do some emotional guarding work before going into a shop. Take a few deep breaths, and visualize a protective golden shield around you. Invisible cloaks work nicely, too. It may sound silly, but the act of wrapping yourself in an imagined cloak is like having a secret power of protection when you need it. Try it. It's fun! Or, if it feels less silly, get an actual cloak or piece of clothing dedicated to invoking feelings of protection around you.

Once you get in the store, take your time and manage your breath. Wait for signals from your inner voice. You may get a sense of "hearing" a stone calling to you, or you may feel "right" when you hold one in your hand. And if you're really just in love with the beauty of one, why not let that beauty move you? Many times, when we want to be more "spiritual," we get confused about what it means and how to proceed. We think that things having to do with beauty are shallow, but that's just another way we are judging ourselves, thus defeating the purpose of being more spiritually centered. If the beauty of a crystal excites you, don't worry if you think you're only picking it because of how it looks. If, when you pick it up and hold it, it feels right, go for it. Being physically attracted to a crystal is just another form of your intuition telling you what you need, and it's just as valid as closing your eyes and relying on feel completely. Be confident in your ability to trust your instincts.

If you're a serious lover of crystals, and I think you just might be, going into a crystal shop can be quite overwhelming! Also, if you're anything like me, you may have to watch your wallet and not take every specimen home with you. It's sometimes helpful to have a clear idea of what kind of crystal you're looking for, and then, if you really feel another one pulling your attention, you can take that as a sign and get that one as well, but this way you'll be entering the environment with a clear objective.

If you purchase your crystals online (see Resources, page 207), you can still use your intuition and feel which one is right for you. Again, use sites that offer plenty of information and have good reviews.

Cleansing Crystals

Crystals store energy, so cleanse them before working with them. Cleansing your crystal can be a special ceremony. When we are working with crystals as representations of aspects of ourselves that we want to nurture, cleansing becomes a way for us to remove the energetic debris we have collected. Removing these particles will help us see ourselves more clearly. Just as everyone picks up emotional baggage through living life, so do crystals. Taking the time to symbolically "wash" away what is no longer necessary should be a common practice for both ourselves and our crystals.

There are many ways to energetically cleanse crystals, so find the way that feels best for you.

- **Brown rice bed:** Arrange a bed of uncooked brown rice on a special plate and rest your crystals on it overnight.

- **Sage:** Light sage and allow the smoke to encompass your crystal. When the smoke envelopes the crystal, it is considered thoroughly cleansed. Use your intuition to determine how long it needs.

- **Visualization:** Imagine a white light pouring through the crystal and see it glowing from the inside out.

- **Sound vibration:** Use instruments with soothing tones, meditation music, or your voice to create sound vibration.

- **Selenite:** Selenite is a crystal that clears the energy of the space it is in. Keeping selenite near your crystals will automatically cleanse their energies.

- **Flower petals and herbs:** Place your crystals on a bed made of flower petals and/or herbs from your garden. Allow them to sit overnight. The leftover flowers and herbs can be used as a soil compost when you're finished.

When working with Chakrubs or yoni eggs, you want to practice good hygiene. Mild natural soap and water is fine for after everyday use. If you wish to disinfect, a bath with a few drops of tea tree oil (melaleuca) and lavender oil is antiviral and antibacterial. Rinse thoroughly with warm water. Always speak to your doctor if you have health concerns, and never push your body to where it's uncomfortable. Every body is different, so make sure it feels right to you.

TIP: When cleansing crystals with water, always make sure you know it is safe for the crystal, as some crystals deteriorate when wet.

The Origins of Sage

Sage is native to countries bordering the Mediterranean Sea and has been celebrated for its culinary and medicinal properties for thousands of years. The Romans treated the plant as sacred and even had a special ceremony for gathering sage. It was used by Greeks and Romans as a preservative for meat, a practice that continued until the beginning of refrigeration and has since been scientifically proven. Its reputation as a healing remedy can be traced back to its scientific name "Salvia officinalis," which is derived from the Latin word *salvere*, meaning "to be saved."

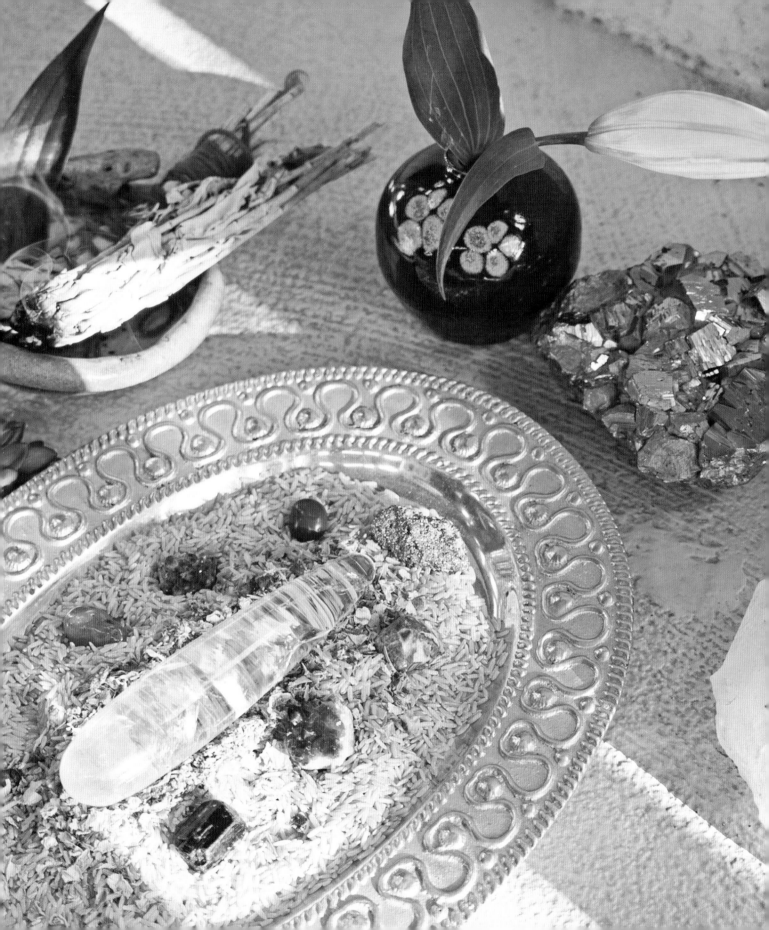

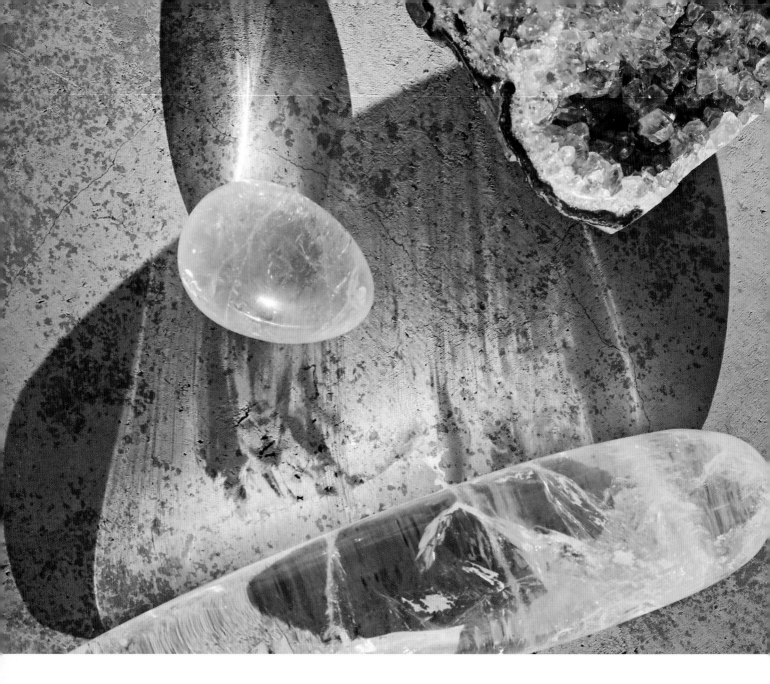

Charging Crystals

Charging crystals is another way to prepare for and enhance your experience when working with them. When you charge a crystal, you are imbuing it with a specific energy and purpose that strengthens your intentions. There are many ways to charge your crystals.

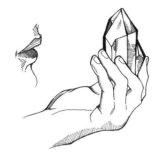

INTENTION

To charge a crystal with a specific intention, find a quiet place to meditate, holding the crystal in your hand. Become clear on your intention for working with it and speak that intention into the crystal.

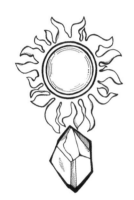

SUNLIGHT

The sun represents masculine, action energy. Placing crystals in the sun is good for when you want to call in active changes. However, crystals such as amethyst, celestite, kunzite, opal, and turquoise may fade in sunlight, so charge them in moonlight instead.

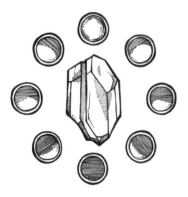

MOONLIGHT

The moon represents feminine, receptive energy. Placing your crystals out to be bathed in moonlight during different phases of the moon allows them to be charged with that energy.

- **New moon:** The new moon occurs when the sun and moon are in alignment, when the masculine energy of the sun merges with the feminine energy of the moon. It represents new beginnings and fresh starts. Charge your crystals under the new moon when you are setting an intention or programming them for a specific use.

- **First quarter:** The waxing quarter moon is a time to look critically at your challenges. You might want to bathe your crystals under this moon phase to call in personal growth or if you are looking for guidance on how to accomplish the intentions set under the new moon.

- **Full moon:** A full moon will be useful when you want to illuminate truths or feel the rewards of everything you have been sowing.

- **Last quarter:** The waning moon is a time to go within and recommit to yourself. Bathe your crystals in this light to nurture your emotions and encourage your intuition.

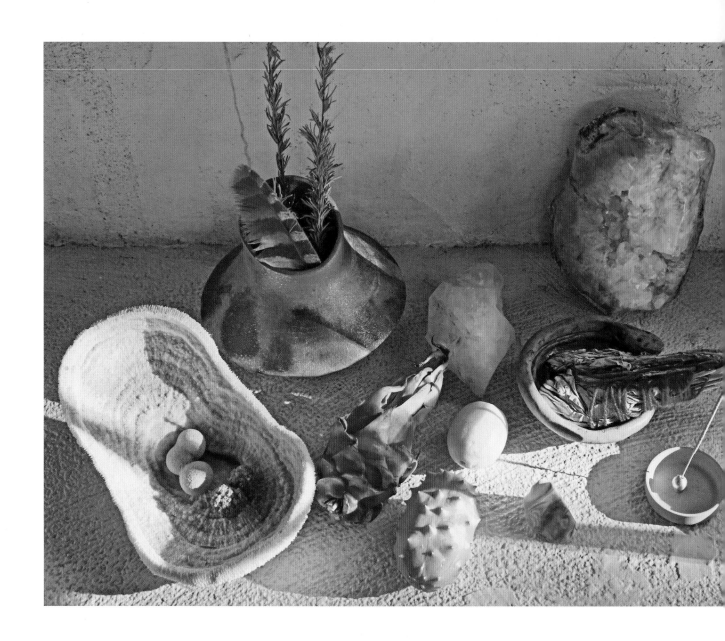

ARRANGING YOUR CRYSTALS AND RITUAL ITEMS ON AN
ALTAR CAN HELP YOU FOCUS ENERGY ON GROUNDING WORK.

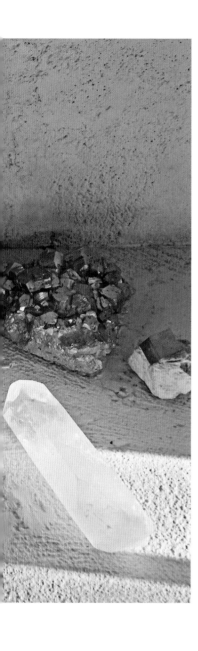

Storing Your Crystals

You may wish to meticulously place crystals around your living area in places that will remind you of your intentions for working with them and to help create beautiful and harmonious feelings in your home. For crystals that you plan to work with often, as in the practices on the following pages, you'll want to create a space that honors both the work and the crystals themselves.

Clear glass display cases are a safe and aesthetic way to store your working crystals. You could also keep the clear box near a window to soak up moon and sun energy through the glass.

Altars are a great way to create a focal point in your living space for your crystals. An altar is a designated area for items that create meaning and focus energy for what is important to you. You can create a theme for your altar to address a specific area of your life, such as pleasure or abundance, or for your specific intentions when going through the practices listed in the following chapters. When creating your altar, choose items that inspire you and reflect your highest self. You might want to add something related to the four natural elements, such as candles to represent fire, seashells to represent water, or something specifically symbolic to your desires. Visit your altar for meditation, journaling, or grounding work. Make sure to clean it every so often and don't be afraid to remove or add items as you evolve.

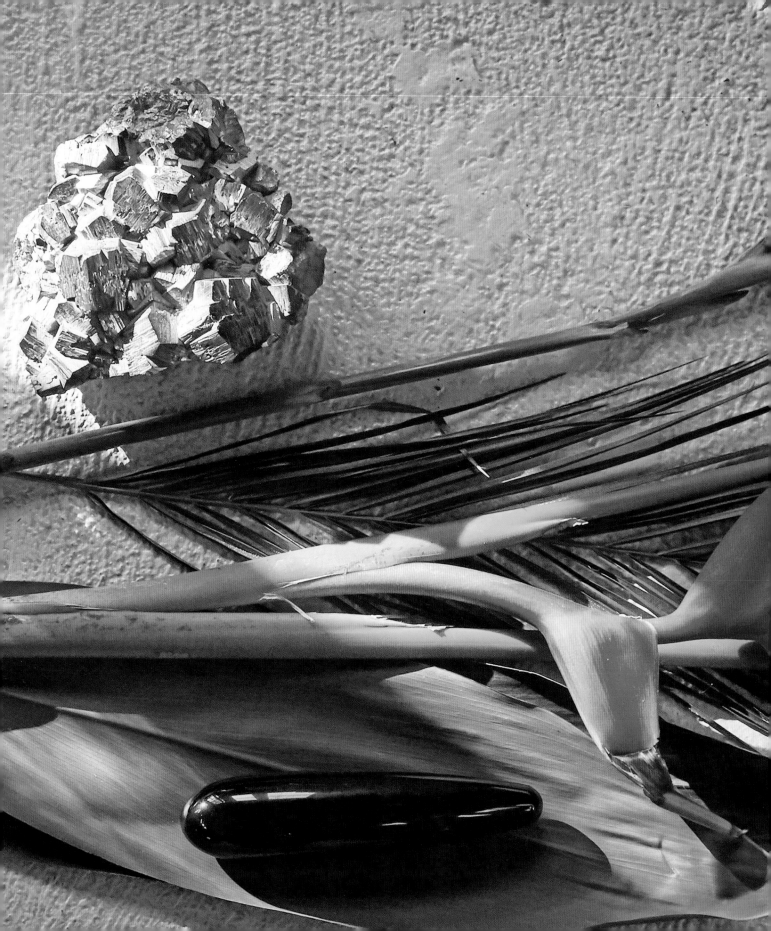

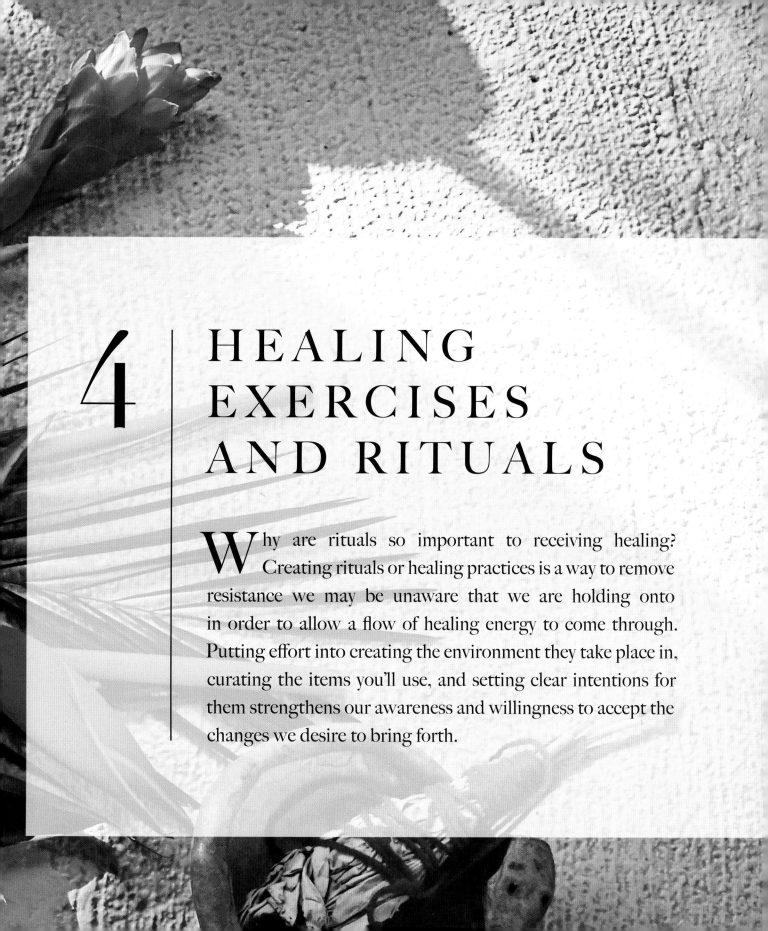

4 | HEALING EXERCISES AND RITUALS

Why are rituals so important to receiving healing? Creating rituals or healing practices is a way to remove resistance we may be unaware that we are holding onto in order to allow a flow of healing energy to come through. Putting effort into creating the environment they take place in, curating the items you'll use, and setting clear intentions for them strengthens our awareness and willingness to accept the changes we desire to bring forth.

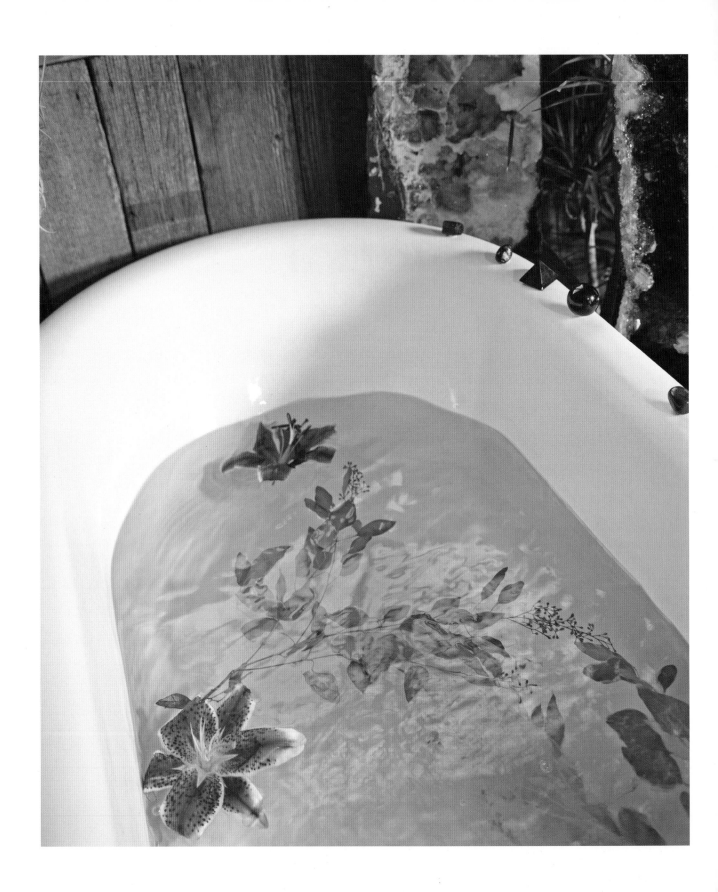

At a time where so much emphasis is put on how we appear to the outside world through social media or otherwise, creating acts meant solely for the purpose of communing with the self in a meaningful and loving way is more valuable now than ever.

It's been proven that the higher our emotional response is to a situation, the more vivid our memory of the event will be. When we practice submitting ourselves and feeling deeply, we are creating more impact within our minds, bringing about more impactful change.

Creating Sacred Space

The act of creating a special and safe environment for yourself is an important element of the work. It's part of the overall recognition that everything has energy and we are affected accordingly. Giving attention to the location you will be occupying for the following exercises sends a signal to your subconscious: This is a space being created for your specific intention. This practice—and you, the beneficiary of this practice—are important and worthy enough to warrant the creation of a special, protected space.

I recommend a clean and quiet area, but it is also okay if it isn't immaculate. If there is laundry that needs folding, or some clutter, use that as a reminder that even in the chaos, there is perfection. The space can be indoors or outdoors, as long as you feel comfortable and know that you will not be disturbed for the length of the exercise.

Cell phones, TVs, computers, and anything connected to Wi-Fi puts invisible electromagnetic smog in our environment. Removing anything transmitting these signals is beneficial when creating a space. Power lines outside our homes also put subtle vibrational disturbances in our environment, but placing crystals in your space specifically for this purpose can disrupt this. If spending time in nature is a natural antidepressant for you, crystals are pieces of nature you can have in your home to support the same effects.

Set Your Intentions

Create a space that's meaningful to you, but don't get caught up in ideas of what being "spiritual" *looks* like. You don't have to wear bohemian-style clothing or trade in handshakes for prayer hands unless they feel authentic to you. When given proper attention, anything you see or experience can be understood as sacred. Opening yourself to the big picture of life enables you to see everything as valuable and meaningful.

Sacred Sex

Sacred sex is typically associated with breathwork and extended periods of eye contact, but other sexual motifs such as discipline and submission can be just as useful for making sacred revelations.

Intention setting is one way to give that necessary attention to a thought, making it sacred. Without necessarily realizing it, we are in a constant state of creation. Because everything is energy, our thoughts and moods affect the world around us. When performing an exercise or ritual, we have a clear space not only in our environment but in our minds to put forth a deliberate intention, as opposed to creating our lives through idle thoughts.

Choose a word, phrase, or visualization to be your intention in these exercises. Depending on what you are inviting to your environment, it could be something like, "I am worthy of the love I receive," or something that resonates with you. Whenever you find yourself losing your focus or getting distracted, come back to your intention. You can chant it like a mantra, or say it silently to yourself. Setting an intention will provide mental clarity as a focal point for when extraneous thoughts or worries pop up. Reminding yourself of how you *want* to feel contributes to making it a reality. If setting an intention feels strange, or as if you are lying to yourself, a simple change can help. In the book *The Amazing Power of Deliberate Intent*, Esther and Jerry Hicks suggest that saying, "Wouldn't it be nice if..." in front of your intention will help bring your vibrational frequency closer to what you are trying to achieve.

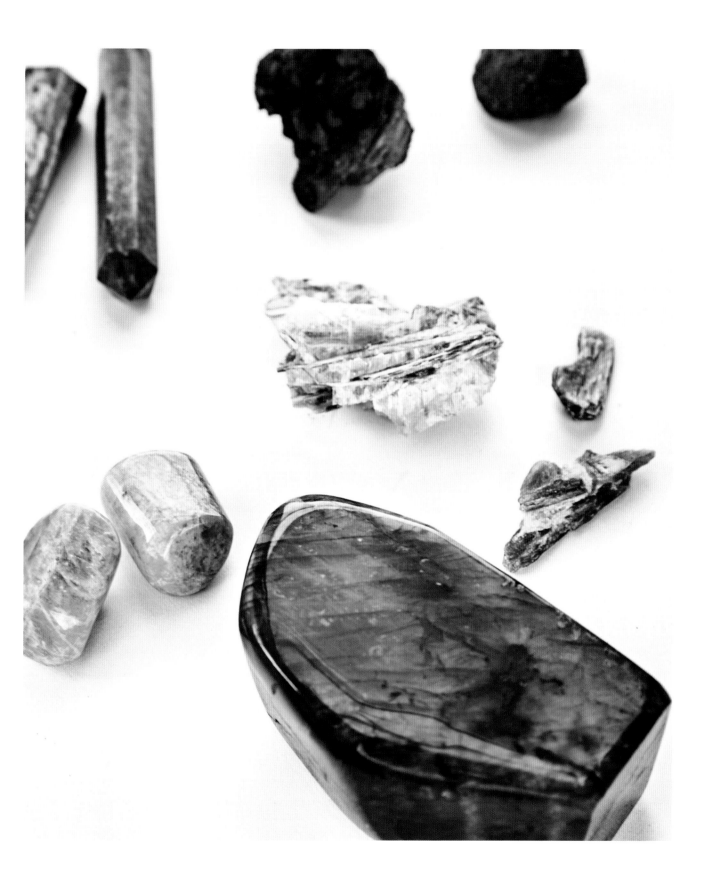

Bringing Yourself

One of the most difficult and most necessary things you'll need to bring to the exercises in this book is simply yourself. Why is it important to gain self-awareness? I've had to ask myself this question a great deal. While creating my brand, I was driven to also understanding the philosophies behind it, which proved to be just as, if not more important, than the products.

Honesty is the path to love. We are dishonest without knowing it, which is why we all hurt each other to some degree, often unintentionally. We are dishonest because we do not yet know who we are. But how could we, unless we give time to evaluate what is important to us, what events have truly shaped us, and what our most important values are?

We can't avoid spending a portion of our lives without knowing who we are. We're meant to get lost, make mistakes, and even fall in love with the people we ultimately know are "wrong" for us. But it's reflecting on these moments that becomes the lifeblood of the rest of our lives. Becoming clear on what we value and why is necessary in developing our self-awareness, which leads to honesty.

If you don't take time to deepen your understanding of who you are, it becomes difficult to receive love. If someone is offering you love but you lack self-awareness, you won't be able to receive that love because you are not being true to yourself. In order to receive the love you are given, you must insist on showing your authentic self. This takes patience, introspection, and dedication, but it is worth it.

Come Naturally

Why do we stay in relationships we know aren't good for us? Why do we eat poorly when we know we should eat healthy? How is it that we know intellectually how to take care of ourselves, yet still make choices against it?

The choices you make all stem from your current state of vibration. To feel in alignment with a decision, your current energy has to resonate with what you choose. Change is difficult because when we tell ourselves we *should* do something, we create a sense of shame. We can have the education and emotional awareness of what is of most value to our lives, but unless we are coming from a place that is inherently choosing to make these healthy choices, they usually won't last.

Instead, what we need to do is find the root of *why* choosing the wrong relationship feels right, or *why* choosing to stay in a job that doesn't fulfill us brings us comfort. When that underlying issue is fixed, doing what is truly healthy for ourselves will feel natural, and that brings about lasting change. Gaining this self-understanding gives you another perspective as you work toward change. Through working with the chakra system and acknowledging the energies at play, and through using crystals to raise vibration to states of health and harmony, the practices in this book address the underlying culprit in making decisions we know aren't aligned with our ultimate well-being: neglecting the needs of our energy field.

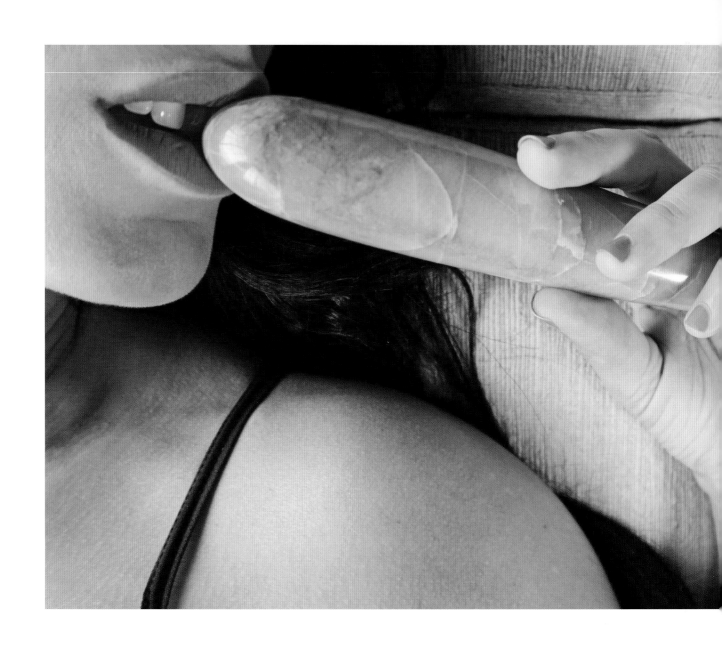

BRING YOUR HONEST SELF AND EMBRACE
YOUR SENSUAL ENERGY.

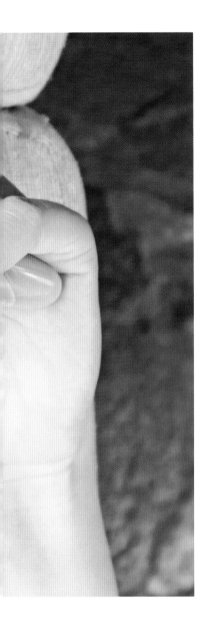

What's Your Style?

Each of us has a different intuitive style that can be further developed by working with our flow of energy. Some people are good at visualization, and others are sensitive to sound. When you discover what type of sensitivity you have, use that as a tool to enhance your experience.

One way to determine your sensitivity is to look at what instinctively turns you on. If visual cues such as erotica turn you on, chances are exercises with visualization will be most beneficial to you. If you are a big fan of dirty talk, introducing sound should be a crucial piece of enhancing your practice. Be it touch, smell, or taste, these are all energy enhancers that can be introduced in each exercise to improve your experience. With repetition and intention, these are muscles that can be strengthened over time. Try different things to see what is most useful for you.

Acting It Out

I spent most of my adolescent life in acting school. Acting at its most fundamental is about the actors willingly changing their energy to achieve a desired performance. A truly gifted actor can access their energy and transform it to fit the scene. It is not just about raising the voice or waving the arms to display anger; it is about evoking that energy from a source of inner power.

While performing the exercises in this book, certain instructions may feel foreign or even silly at first. But by "acting" like you feel the energy of your chakras and the crystals, you create the space to *actually* feel them.

When a skilled actor is performing a scene in which he needs to convey joy or sadness, he will often look for ways in which to actually conjure up this emotion. It is the same principle when it comes to increasing positive energy in your body. You have the resources within you to bring forth what you want to feel, and sometimes a "fake it 'till you make it" attitude is helpful.

Just as an actor does, when you perform an exercise you are reciting the script, being aware of the movements, and bringing up energy that is necessary to experience the objective and make it feel authentic. The better an actor knows the script and blocking, the easier it is to find the essence of the mission of the scene. Just as an actor rehearses to accomplish this, read through the exercises ahead of time and prepare yourself to get started.

Grant Yourself Consent

Before performing any of the self-love practices, create a dialogue with yourself to make sure you feel open to receiving and giving yourself this intimate attention. This creates a bond with your body and your intentions and helps strengthen the trust you have with yourself. Many of us engage in sexual activity before we comprehend the powerful energy that plays a part in it. Learning to consent with ourselves and making sure we are honoring our own boundaries is important for deepening our self-love.

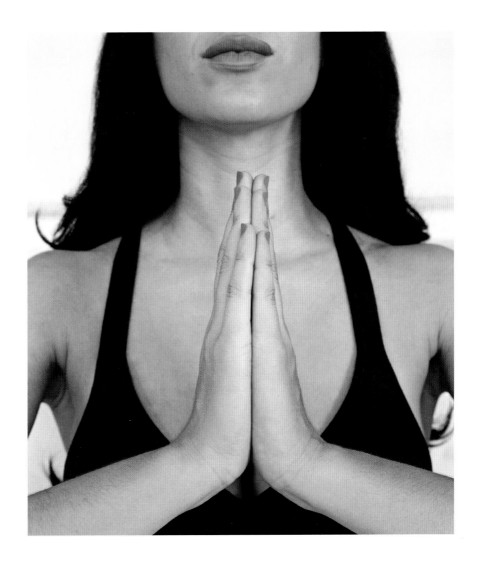

ASK FOR AND GRANT YOURSELF CONSENT
TO EMBRACE SELF-LOVE.

All these exercises can be modified to fit your needs. For example, you may decide not to practice sexual touching and instead focus on the breath and tuning in to your crystal. Listen to yourself and what is right for you. Sometimes it may be right to nudge yourself toward trying something new, and other times it may be right to be patient with yourself as you open to this type of healing. There is no wrong choice here.

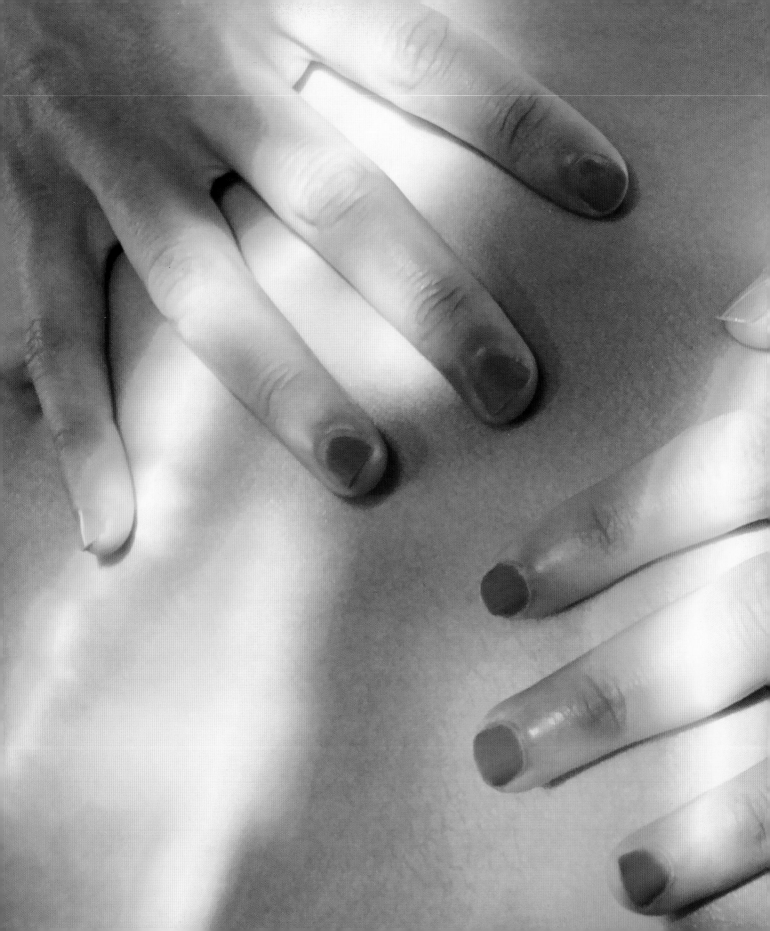

5 | INVITING SELF-LOVE

We are all children of the earth, comprised of the same minerals found throughout nature. There are even crystals in our bones—crystalline structures are in our skeletal structure, our teeth, and in our ears. Without anything else, you can tap into this crystalline energy and remind yourself that you already possess the tools you require for any journey you set foot on. Crystals help facilitate our natural ability to heal, but it is *you* who heals you. Different crystals will bring out different energies, but it is all within you.

Somewhere along the line, we downplay our divinity. We're taught to follow rules instead of our intuition. We begin to question our authority over our lives and lose our sense of co-creation with the universe. To benefit from all that crystals have to offer you, it is important to remind yourself that you are a powerful being.

The body is where we start. You must understand the magnificence you are walking around with all day, and to do that we explore self-love.

Masturbation as a Symbol of Self Love

When I say masturbation, I do not just mean genital play. *Self-pleasure* is the better term, because it involves anything you do to create a more loving relationship with yourself, through touch or loving thoughts. For example, I have some nervous habits—I pick at my skin or pinch myself when I'm feeling anxious. The best way I've found to stop myself is to repeat the phrase, "I love you" to myself when it happens. It may seem silly at first, but it is hard to do self-destructive acts when you're being given love.

When approached from a healthy perspective, masturbation can be experienced as an act of pure love. Coupled with the intention of creating positive culminations, it can be a gesture that evokes feelings of safety, body positivity, and comfort. We are creating energy within our bodies when we give ourselves pleasure. That energy becomes fuel for us when we learn how to channel it.

From a practical standpoint, orgasms are good for your health and have been proven to reduce depression and stress, regulate the immune system, increase fertility, and lower blood pressure. When we honor our ability to soothe ourselves and see pleasure as a gift bestowed upon us, we can begin to cultivate the very transcendental emotion of gratitude.

Becoming "stuck" in certain sexual fantasies, acts, or habits, such as self-pleasuring the same way each time or needing a specific fantasy to "get off," is a signal that there may be an energy blockage. When you recognize an energy blockage, you can try to understand what has caused it and then move it.

Holding on to a sexual fantasy can be a sign that a correlating chakra is weak. This does not mean it's bad—we all have kinks, and that is natural, normal, and fun. But it can signify an energy block when you are stuck on a fantasy or cannot enjoy sex without going to a specific idea. When that block is accepted and released, you can enjoy the full potential of your sexuality, which will permeate your everyday life.

For example, when a sexual fantasy becomes a recurring part of your self-pleasuring sessions, take note of why its aspects turn you on and what they symbolize. Fantasizing about having someone take control over you, for example, could indicate an underlying desire to surrender. It could be a signal to "let go" more often in your daily life to satisfy your need to trust in the universe. Working with turquoise and generally most blue crystals can promote a vibration of universal trust. Chrysanthemum stone is also said to bring about an understanding of the bigger picture in life, which allows for a trusting attitude.

It may not be fun to examine why you've become dependent on your sexual habits or fantasies. And you'll always have specific kinks that turn you on, but when they become a crutch, take it as a sign that there is an energetic block you need to release.

Each ritual is a journey in itself. Come back to these rituals again and again. Allow your experiences to differ and explore possibilities within yourself and your own internal healing. See the instructions as suggestions and feel free to adjust them accordingly. These are meant to be gentle exercises with the ability to expand as deeply as you wish to go.

Treasure Within Exercise

This exercise is an easy way to include self-love practices in your everyday routine. It combines crystal healing, self-massage, and the therapeutic art of eye-gazing. It only adds 5 to 7 minutes to your daily routine (but can last longer, if you would like!). Keeping a crystal charged with your intention on your bathroom counter can help act as a reminder to include this practice in your daily routine.

Have you ever looked into your own eyes? It may feel strange at first, but the more you do it, the easier it becomes. Before getting into the shower, take some time looking into the mirror. Focus on your eyes. There is a reason why they say eyes are the windows to the soul. Looking into someone's eyes or into your own eyes for an extended period can be a spiritual experience in itself. It is a bonding and trust building exercise.

1. Place one or both hands on your heart in front of the mirror.

2. Close your eyes and take a deep breath in. As you exhale, open your eyes.

3. Gaze softly into your less dominant eye.

4. Try to keep a steady focus, and imagine you are looking deeper and deeper within the eye.

5. Tell yourself aloud or silently: "Thank you for seeing me for who I really am. I love you, I forgive you, and to continue this love I will..." Finish the thought.

6. Step into the shower.

Materials

· Mirror
· Shower

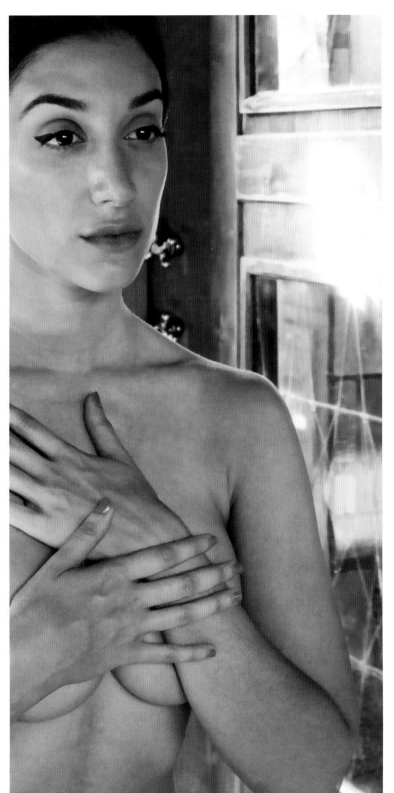

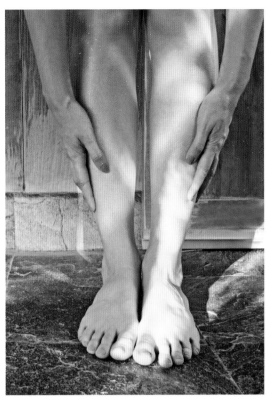

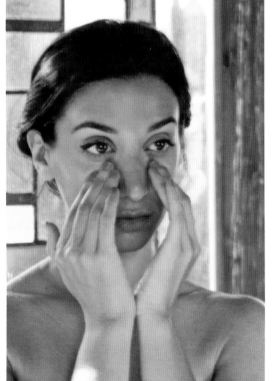

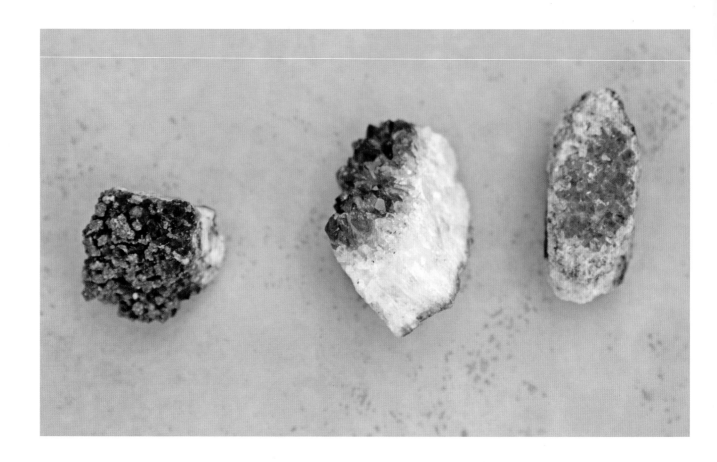

KEEP A CRYSTAL CHARGED WITH YOUR INTENTION
ON THE BATHROOM COUNTER AS A REMINDER TO
PRACTICE SELF-LOVE.

7. In the shower, recognize that within you there is crystal. Imagine that the shower has acted as a cleansing agent, just like you would use to clear any other crystals (see page 71). Tune in to what you feel a crystal goes through energetically when it is being cleaned. Feel excess and unnecessary energy running off you, down into the shower drain.

8. After the shower, once you get out and while still wet, take a deep breath and imagine your skeleton inside you, glowing with the crystals throughout.

9. State this intention: "I appreciate all my body does for me."

10. Rub your hands together so they become warm. Now, put your focus on your toes—you may touch them if you'd like. With your attention, you are activating this part of you. This can be done by imagining orgasmic energy but placing it in your toes. Focus your attention on the bones in all your little toes, and feel the subtle vibration of the crystals within you. Give thanks to this part of your body.

11. Move up toward every part of you, thinking deep down all the way through to the skeletal system. Keep imagining the orgasmic energy moving to each part of the body you focus on. How does it feel to caress and give praise to every inch of you? How does it feel to know of the inner workings that are happening constantly within you?

12. Keep doing this while working all the way up to your facial structure. Softly caress your face with the tips of your fingers. You are creating a circuit of enhanced energy, simply by putting your attention on these underlying minerals within you.

13. To finish, stand erect. Take deep breaths and smile (your teeth have crystal, too!). Acknowledge the positive choices you have made to give yourself loving attention. Doing this exercise often will benefit the relationship you have with yourself, by putting emphasis on the way you feel inside of your body.

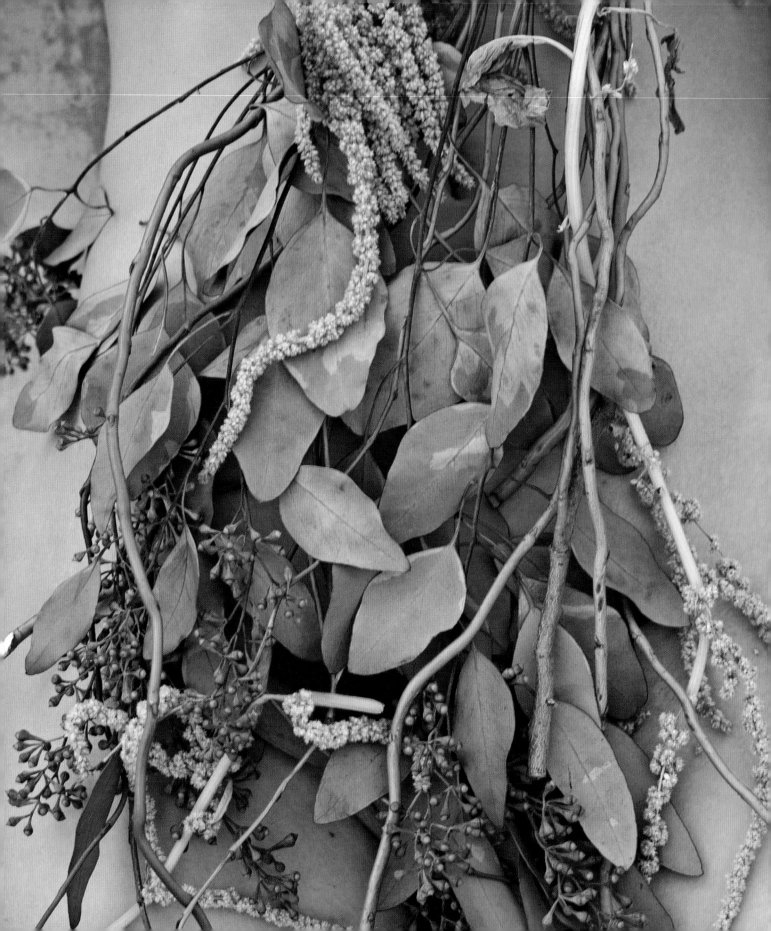

6 | THE ROOT CHAKRA

The root chakra, located at the base of the spine, is the seat of Kundalini energy. *Kundalini* comes from the Sanskrit word *kundal*, which means "coil" or "spiral." You can picture Kundalini energy as a coiled, sleeping snake, or two inter-coiled snakes, that lies at the root chakra and awakens through awareness and intention. Visualizing these snakes climbing up the spine as sexual energy moves up the chakras can even enhance pleasure.

Many books have been written on raising Kundalini energy. Some even come with a warning, as raising Kundalini before you are emotionally and spiritually ready is not recommended.

The root chakra manages our immune system in a general sense, the lower extremities, our hips, the rectum, genitalia such as the vagina, and the elimination system. It is also associated with the adrenal gland, which manages stress and our sense of "fight or flight."

The energy of the root chakra is that of the Divine Mother. Because it shares space with our genitals, we reacquaint ourselves with where we all come from—the heavenly birthing place and home—when we spend time in this area. When we connect to the energy field of this chakra, we connect to the divine portal that brought us to earth.

Root Chakra Snapshot

Color: Soft pink to deep blood red

Secondary Color: Black

Sensual Sound: *Uh*

Musical Tone: C

Location: Base of spine

Governs: Physical sensation, keeping you grounded, physical survival, instincts

Healthy: Positive self-image, energy, stamina, confidence

Unhealthy: Insecure, all sexual stimulation in genitals, not grounded, uncertain

Sense: Smell

Organ: Nose

Sexuality: Primal, basic instincts

Element: Earth

Intention: I Am

A Healthy Root Chakra

Word Origin: Root Chakra

All our knowledge regarding the chakras draws from ancient tantric Hinduism. The Sanskrit word for the root chakra is *muladhara*. *Mula* means "root" and *adhara* means "support" or "base."

The root chakra is responsible for our sense of safety and security; it's connected to our ability to provide for basic needs such as food, water, and shelter. It grounds us and governs our ability to integrate into the physical world. A healthy root chakra provides a foundation for energy to move through the rest of the chakra system.

When our root chakra is pure and functioning at its full potential, we feel worthy of pleasure and love. We are connected to our place in the world because we link to the strength of our ancestors and our spiritual path. We call upon our root chakra when we summon courage, resourcefulness, and resilience.

A fully functioning root chakra gives us confidence in our sexual identity. It helps us to achieve a healthy sexual appetite with firm boundaries and a sense of safety. It also influences who you may be attracted to, since this chakra governs the sense of smell. Primal attraction is heavily influenced by scent: Through sense of smell, you pick up on pheromones, a chemical released as a subconscious sex signal which affects the attractiveness of a mate.

When the Root Chakra Needs Acknowledgment

Because our root chakra is so closely tied to our basic survival instincts, it is easy to recognize when there is a blockage in its region. We store early childhood traumas, even trauma from being birthed, in our root chakra. Abandonment issues and sexual abuse may also cause blockages here, leading to feelings of instability, lack of boundaries, and shamefulness.

Symptoms of a blocked root chakra include lack of energy or motivation, being irritable for seemingly no reason, and feeling disconnected from the physical world. There may be energy stuck in this area if a person's sexual experience is purely genital, meaning orgasms are restricted to the groin as opposed to full body sensations. When this energy is not processed, it often leads to impulsive sexual behavior that we later regret. Alternatively, there may be a block if someone has closed themselves off from sex completely. This is different from being asexual; not a preference, this is when your relationship to sex has changed. Difficulty achieving orgasm may also indicate a blocked root chakra.

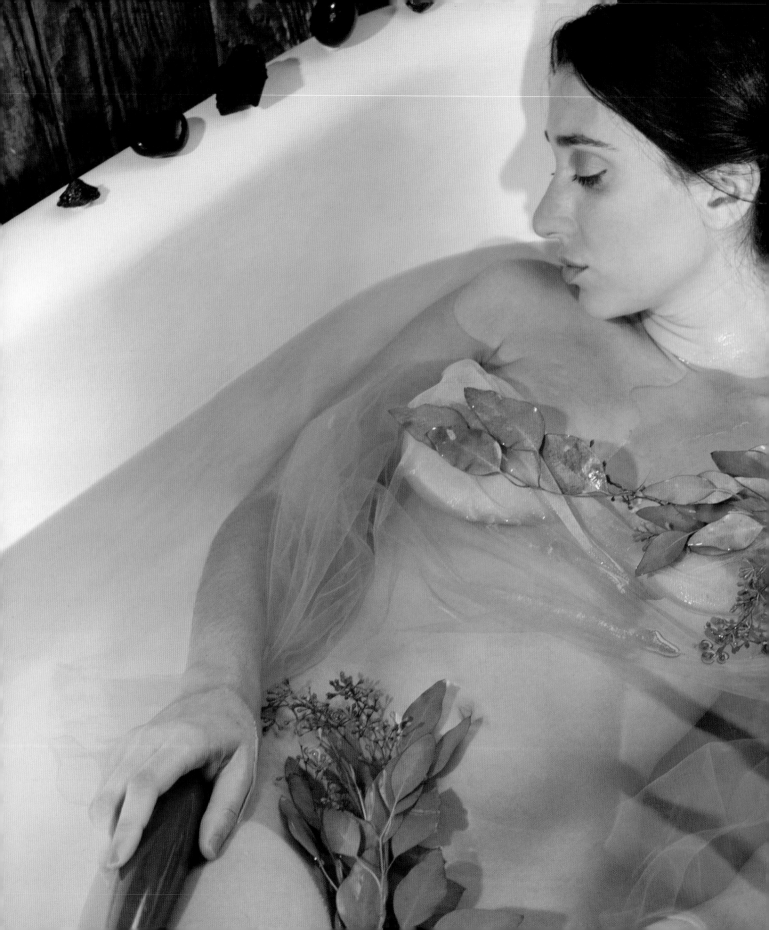

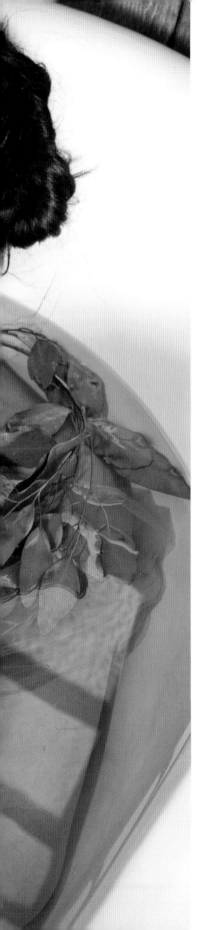

Revising My Understanding of Self-Pleasure

When I was about six years old, I was walking around the pool while my mother cleaned it. I was casually caressing my chest when she yelled, "Stop that! Stop doing that right now!" I felt immediate shame for innocently touching my chest area, a place that to me was no different from my elbow.

Another time, my family was watching a movie where the lead actors shared a passionate kiss. When my sisters and I exclaimed, "Ewwww!" in response, our mother gave us a lecture us on the beauty of this expression of love.

Without knowing it at the time, I was being conditioned to believe that pleasure when romance was involved was acceptable, but pleasure for pleasure's sake was not. I was too young at the time to understand how to process these feelings, which weren't inherently mine. Even so, they remained my beliefs about pleasure until I made the conscious decision to release them.

How Sexuality Is Learned

Before we know what sexuality really is, we are exposed to projections our elders have concerning the subject. Before many of us hit puberty, we learn about sex consciously and subconsciously. It is critical to stop and take the time to understand our deep-seated values and the causes for our sexual behavior, because we are often guided by the beliefs of our elders projected onto us before we had the wisdom to reject their philosophies.

Spend some time considering your personal beliefs when it comes to sexuality and pleasure. Can you decipher which ones stem from your own value system and which ones were passed down by people who raised you, members of your community, or entertainment sources? Ask yourself these questions and give yourself the freedom to let go of anything that does not serve your journey.

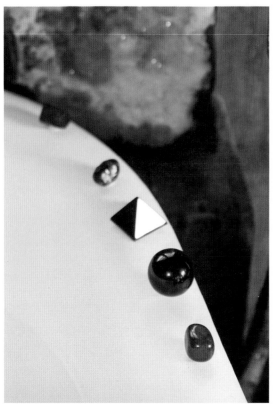

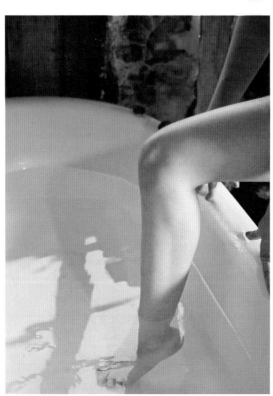

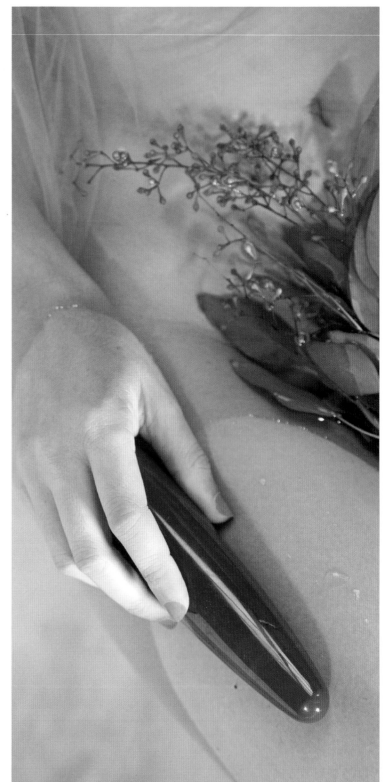

The Lotus Grows Out of the Mud:
ROOT CHAKRA RITUAL

Just as the lotus flower blooms in the least likely of physical environments, we have the ability to transform our deepest pain into opportunities for growth.

To truly relax and achieve release, find a place where you can feel completely comfortable and free from distraction. Create a sacred, safe space where you can unleash everything that you have been holding in. An ideal place to "tune in" and focus on self-care for this exercise is the bathtub, but if a bathtub is unavailable for you, you can perform the same ritual in any comfortable space and visualize the water aspects of this exercise.

The root chakra, greatly associated with the genitals, can connect us to the innocence of discovering our pleasure bodies. Revitalizing this chakra enables us to rebirth ourselves so that we feel safe and worthy in our exploration and discovery of pleasure. We tap into feelings of giving birth to ourselves, while also experiencing this energy as the child, feeling protected and giving ourselves unconditional love.

To focus on your root chakra and ignite its energy, this exercise will help you honor one of your most basic primal instincts: seeking pleasure. The pleasure you will be exploring here will come from labia massage. The labia are often ignored, so giving them attention can be soothing and beneficial. The outer labia typically grow more hair than the inner labia and are less sensitive than the inner labia. Everybody's labia are different; some are thick and plump while others are slender. The inner labia are typically not covered by hair but are different on everyone. Some inner labia can be longer than the outer labia, they can be different on either side, and they can be pink or deep purple. This is a more sensitive erogenous zone as through massaging it will lead to touching the clitoris.

TIP: If you don't have a vulva, you can vary this exercise to focus on building energy in the root chakra area of the body.

Set an Intention

Think of your intention as an anchor in your practice. Whenever you find yourself losing your focus or getting distracted, come back to your intention. It can be a word, a phrase, or even a visualization. You can chant it like a mantra, or say it silently to yourself. You may also choose to repeat the sensual sound related to the root chakra, which is a deep and drawn-out "uh" sound.

Choose Your Crystals

Choose black crystals such as tourmaline, onyx, or obsidian, or any crystal that gives you a sense of safety. You will also want to keep red jasper, bloodstone, or another red crystal handy. See detailed crystal descriptions on page 108.

See detailed crystal descriptions on page 108.

Materials

· Crystal(s)

· Bathtub (If you don't have a tub, imagine you are in a body of water.)

1.   Place the black crystals in a circle around you or the perimeter of a tub, signifying safety.

2.   Undress, get in a warm bath, and begin by taking several deep breaths.

3.   Create an intention for this practice to help you focus on the ideas, memories, and feelings you need to release. If you aren't sure what they are, your intention might be to release emotions, ideas that no longer serve you, memories that keep you in the past, or energetic ties to unhealthy relationships.

4.   Massage where your inner thighs and vulva meet in circular motions with your fingertips.

5.   Move to massaging one side of your outer labia, starting at the top in circular motions, moving all the way down. Lightly squeeze, tickle, and experiment with different amounts of pleasure. Repeat on the other side.

6.   Try "rolling" up the labia to create a gentle pressure around the clitoris with all four fingertips on each hand. Roll, stretch. Go with what is most enjoyable to you. Remember to take your time.

7.   In this space you have created, you may release memories or ideas as sexual energy builds. Continue to breathe deeply and know that the circle of crystals you've created offers you protection.

8.   Take note of what feelings or sensations arise and, when they do, acknowledge them, breathe deeply, and continue.

9.   When you feel ready, continue with gentle touch on the inner labia.

10. Start on one side, gently pressing with your fingers and moving from the top to the bottom. Lightly squeeze, tickle, and experiment with different amounts of pleasure. Move to the other side.

11. Keep breathing and continue for at least five minutes.

You may continue for as long as you'd like, and you may even achieve orgasm, but an orgasm is not necessary. At the close of this massage, state your intention aloud: "I release that which is not useful to my greatest good." Take a few more moments to live in the water with all the energy you just conjured.

Allow the water to drain while envisioning everything you don't need being given back to the earth to transmute into something different. Take the red crystal in your left hand, and rinse off with cool water.

As you dry off, imagine that you're removing any residue of negative energies or thoughts you sent down the drain. Relax in bed while holding the red crystal near your root chakra. Imagine the energy from the crystal replenishing your root chakra with its energy. Visualize the crystal within your root chakra, filling it with its powerful red vibrancy. To end this practice, you can choose to fall asleep, to bring your hands together in prayer and give gratitude to yourself, or to journal about your experience.

Extras for the Root Chakra

Because root chakra is associated with the sense of smell, aromatherapy is a powerful addition to this exercise. The essential oils closely associated with the root chakra tend to be made of heavier molecules and are characterized as base notes, which are deeper, slowly unfolding, long-lasting scents. These include:

Angelica *(Angelica archangelica)*

Cedar, Atlantic *(Cedrus altantica)*

Cedar, Himalayan *(Cedrus deodora)*

Frankincense *(Boswellia carteri)*

Linden Blossom *(Tilia vulgares* or *T. europeae)*

Myrrh *(Commiphora myrrha)*

Patchouli *(Pogostemon cablin)*

Spikenard *(Nardostachys jatamansi)*

Vetiver *(Vetiveria zizanoides)*

Crystals for the Root Chakra

To work with your root chakra, first use a black crystal to release and then a red crystal to replenish. Black is the color of the unknown, and we often associate its heavy energy with negative elements. Black stones can help you reclaim your power and shield you from harm. They strengthen your sense of security and enhance psychic abilities while keeping you grounded.

As the color that is reflected in blood and fire, red has a strong energy. It is full of passion and life force, and it invokes masculine energy. Dark red crystals can increase motivation and devotion, helping us communicate deep feelings. Here is a list of some of my favorites to use. Choose ones that speak to you on a personal level. Listen to your intuition.

Black Obsidian

When volcanic lava cools rapidly with minimal crystallization, black obsidian is formed. Once used as the material for ancient mirrors, they reveal our shadow selves. This intense energy is often labeled as "negative," but black obsidian has the potential to help us confront our demons and release mental stress while offering protection. Its edge is thinner and sharper than high-quality surgical steel and it is used in today's scalpels for the most precise surgery.

BENEFITS:

Eases past relationship trauma and overcoming emotional strain

— Creates emotional stability

— Assists in past life healing and can resolve issues related to previous misuse of power

— Assists in learning and implementing self-control

— Helps to overcome stress

— Promotes clarity when making difficult decisions

— Promotes positive sexual health and easing the root chakra, ovaries, womb, and menses

Black Tourmaline

Black tourmaline is a protection stone that provides a psychic shield to repel and dispel negative energies, entities, or destructive forces. When charged, one end becomes positive and the other negative, allowing the stone to attract or repel particles of dust. It was once used by Dutch traders in the 1700s to pull ash from their Meerschaum pipes.

BENEFITS:

Guards against environmental pollutants

— Purifies and neutralizes negative thoughts and internal conflicts, transforming them into productive, positive energy

— Grounds and restores your connection to the earth

— Promotes a sense of self-confidence and empowerment

— Reduces anxiety and stress

— Provides protection during ritual work

— Relieves insecurities around unworthiness

— Strengthens the sense of smell and enhances response to pheromones

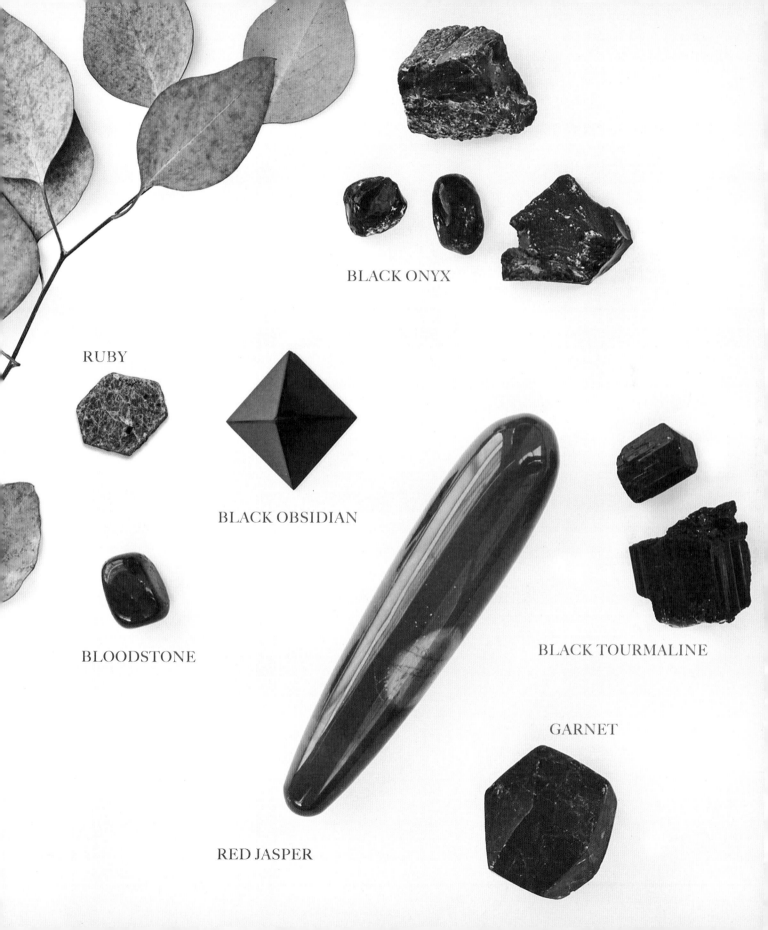

BLACK ONYX

RUBY

BLACK OBSIDIAN

BLACK TOURMALINE

BLOODSTONE

GARNET

RED JASPER

Black Onyx

Described in the first book of the Bible as an element of creation, black onyx was equally revered and feared in ancient cultures. Some thought it to be a symbol of bad luck that caused sadness and depression and brewed discord between family members and lovers. Over time practitioners were able to harness this dark energy and use it for good.

BENEFITS:

Grounds, protects against, and eliminates excess or unwanted energies

— Increases stamina and self-control

— Releases difficult emotions such as sorrow and grief

— Sharpens your senses

— Increases self-confidence and responsibility

— Provides strength to end unhappy relationships

— Promotes a healthy sense of self

— Deflects negative thoughts and criticism from others and defends against manipulation

— Provides physical strength and builds character

— Brings stability to marriage and partnerships

Red Jasper

Associated in ancient Egyptian cultures with the fertilizing blood of Mother Isis, red jasper supports the circulatory system ad detoxifies the blood. It carries a strong spiritual grounding vibration and creates a strong connection to the earth. It is a stone of passion that is sometimes used as a token to consummate love.

BENEFITS:

Nurtures and heals the spirit while increasing courage and wisdom

— Encourages focus, self-control, and mastery

— Enhances tantric sex

— Assists in identifying personal beliefs about sexual expression and/or orientation and helps release related shame or guilt

— Can assist in overcoming resistance to committed relationships or jealousy

— Injects freshness and new ideas into creative work

— Beneficial for performers and helps them be more sensitive to their audience

— Raises Kundalini energy

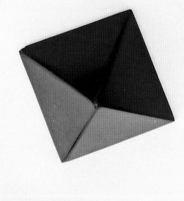

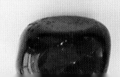

Garnet

Garnet honors Sekhmet, the Egyptian Goddess of war and healing. It is thought to enhance strength and has been worn for centuries as a talisman of protection. It helps bring stability to chaos and can be used to release bad karma.

BENEFITS:

Offers protection from evil, nightmares, and during travel

— Useful for accessing ancestral memories and used by medicine men to cure depression

— Stimulates Kundalini energy and aids sexual potency

— Aids in emotional recovery and rebuilding the spirit

— Enhances intuition and encourages spiritual growth

— Sharpens perception of the self and others

— Promotes a balanced approach to sensuality, sexuality, and intimacy

— Prevents fear and insecurity

Bloodstone

Legend claims that bloodstone was first formed when the blood of Jesus Christ met the earth and turned to stone. Its associations with blood and circulation have persisted throughout ancient cultures to present day. Bloodstone lends support during adverse times and calms the emotional body.

BENEFITS:

Provides support to women during their childbearing years and beyond by easing the birthing process, alleviating symptoms associated with menstruation, and stabilizing hormones for those approaching menopause

— Provides emotional support and clarity during times of extreme adversity

— Offers support to those who have been bullied or abandoned

— Gives wisdom to know when to withdraw from volatile situations

— Provides centering and grounding amidst chaos

— Dispels confusion and enhances decision-making, self-confidence, and self-sufficiency

— Increases adaptability and organization

— Reduces confusion, stress, and anxiety

— Helps release emotional trauma and guilt

— Brings abundance, success, and prosperity

Ruby

Natural ruby is one of four "precious" gemstones (along with diamond, emerald, and sapphire) known for its rarity, monetary value, and hardness (second only to diamond). Ruby encourages a healthy passion for life and allows us to move past pain to share love with others.

BENEFITS:

Fosters peace and drives away frightful dreams while restraining lust, and resolving disputes

— Supports blood and the circulatory system, and can regulate menstrual flow and relieve associated pain

— Used for treatment of sexual dysfunction, impotence, infertility, and early menopause

— Encourages healing from pain and transmutes negative energy and anger

— Provides strength to release victimhood and encourages a more positive and courageous outlook

— Increases desire and sexual energy and can be used to activate Kundalini energy

— Associated with faithful passion, commitment, and intimacy

— Helps develop a healthy self-esteem and overcome insecurities related to feeling ugly or unloved

— Encourages one to stand up for others and speak out against wrongs committed to children, friends, family, or the environment

— Encourages one to follow their bliss

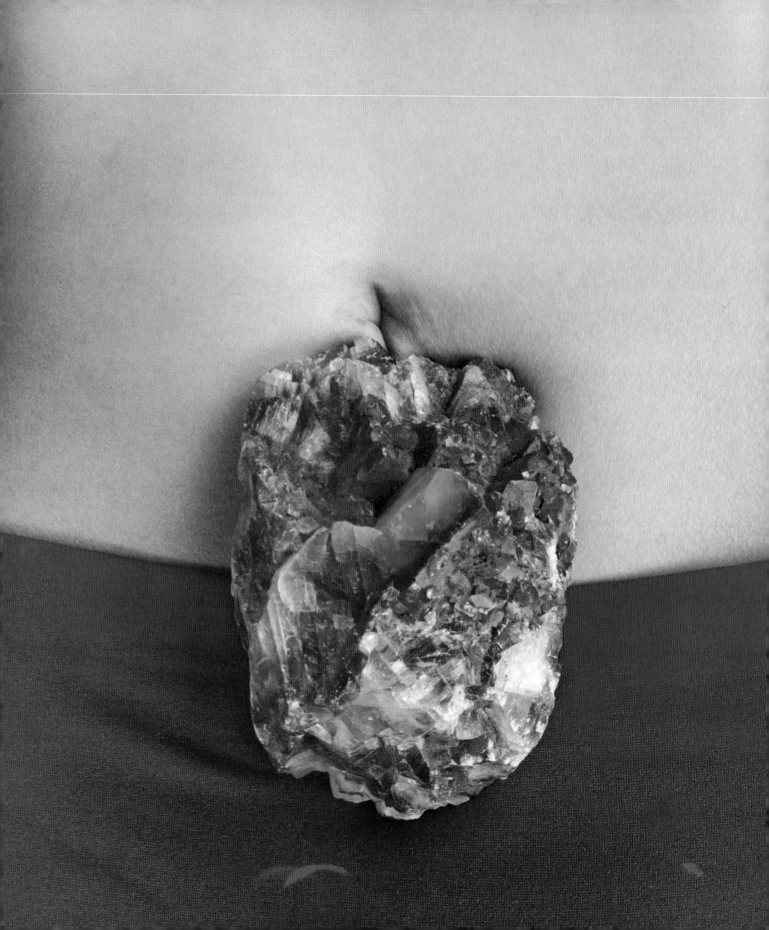

7 | THE SACRAL/ SEX CHAKRA

The sacral or sex chakra's symbolism relates to water energy, bringing nourishment and sweetness through exchange with those we love. It is associated with the lumbosacral nerve plexus and the gonads (the testes for male bodies and ovaries for female bodies). The pelvic area is also governed by this chakra.

As an archetype energy, the sex chakra is that of the Emperor/Empress. With it, we learn to take pleasure in what physical life has to offer, and we learn to feel worthy of its gifts. We learn the art of sacred indulgence while staying in touch with integrity, releasing guilt for whatever goodness we experience. The sacral chakra shows us that our bodies are vessels in which our spirits may explore the physical realm. This awareness lets us take pleasure in anything "human" we experience in our lives, giving us an appreciation not only for what feels good but for anything that alerts us to the reality of our bodies and emotions. When we feel sorrow, we appreciate it for the depth it is creating in our soul. When we feel pain, we appreciate it for the reminder that we are alive.

The sacral chakra is associated with taste but teaches us how to indulge in all the senses. Nourishing it helps us mindfully connect to all those senses, providing a deep gratitude for experiencing life through sight, smell, taste, sound, and touch.

The sacral chakra governs our emotional relationships to ourselves and to others. It allows us to feel passionate about life, bringing an awareness of the pleasure it is to be human. Because we appreciate ourselves as beings, we are able to see others in this light as well. Connecting to this chakra allows us to take pleasure in other people's pleasure—a true key to fulfillment. When your sacral chakra is functioning in full health, you relate to everything with a sense of full connection. You feel empathetic, and you find it easy to be present and revel in the moment when receiving and giving sexual pleasure.

The sacral chakra rules our emotions, our creativity, and our sensuality. This is where our creativity resides. It is in tune with our creative force and our drive to create through feelings of connection and bondedness. The sacral and throat chakras are connected, as the throat chakra is what provides us the willingness to express our creativity. With a healthy sacral chakra, we can receive pleasure by providing pleasure, and we can understand that we provide pleasure through receiving.

Sex Chakra Snapshot

<u>Color</u>: Pale peach to deep orange

<u>Sensual Sound</u>: *Oo*

<u>Musical Tone</u>: D

<u>Location</u>: 1 to 2 inches (2.5 to 5 cm) below the navel

<u>Governs</u>: Uterus, vagina, cervix, pelvis

<u>Healthy</u>: Fluidity, emotional intelligence, vitality, sexual satisfaction, compassion, bonding

<u>Unhealthy</u>: Guilty about sex, fearful, overly sensitive, rigidity of body and of beliefs, lack of social skills

<u>Sense</u>: Taste

<u>Organ</u>: Tongue

<u>Sexuality</u>: Giving and receiving sexual pleasure, reproduction

<u>Element</u>: Water

<u>Intention</u>: I Feel

A Healthy Sacral Chakra

When balanced and open, a healthy sacral chakra will make it easy to connect and form bonds with others and to feel naturally confident and outgoing. This chakra, when functioning properly, allows one to acknowledge others without envy and take joy in others' free expression of their best selves. There is a presence of vitality in a person who is healthy in this center—someone with a general sensuality due to the ability to take pleasure in the little things. Sexual expression is conveyed with intense sensuality. This sensuality spills over into areas of life not just pertaining to sex but including everyday activities such as washing your face or eating breakfast.

When the Sacral Chakra Needs Acknowledgment

Word Origin: Sex Chakra

The Sanskrit word for this chakra is *svadhisthana*, meaning "the dwelling place of the self." *Sva* means "self" and *adhisthana* means "dwelling place" or "home."

A common trauma associated with the sacral chakra is the lack of nurturing touch in childhood. Just as the root chakra highlights our primal need for sex in terms of procreation, the sacral chakra highlights the need for touch for touch's sake. Affection is a necessity just like food or water. Arousal, just like hunger or thirst, can act as a signal that we are craving intimacy, that it is time to acknowledge our need for affection.

Rather than seeing arousal as an annoyance, like a headache you want to get rid of by taking medicine, try to see it as a call to action to bring more attention to yourself or a creative idea that you may be ignoring.

When this chakra is deficient in energy, sex becomes predominantly about orgasmic release and not about bonding or emotional connection; it signifies that energy is stagnant in the root chakra. Learning to move energy upward into the sacral chakra prevents sexuality from staying in a primitive state. Frigid bodies and beliefs, fear of change, and lack of desire are signifiers of a deficient sacral chakra energy.

If this chakra is in excess, addictions may arise. They may be addictions to sex, to romance, or to emotionally high and low relationships. A poorly functioning sacral chakra may be indicated by co-dependency and/or manipulation through seduction. Someone with an unhealthy sacral chakra has a sense of detachment that may come across to others as immaturity in relationships. In people with predominantly masculine energies, the sacral chakra can become damaged when the person is taught dysfunctional ideas about sexuality, pleasure, or emotion.

The Sacral Chakra and Spirituality

It is through the sacral chakra that I strengthened my idea of spirituality. Spirituality to me is being aware that you were here before you were born and that you will still exist after you die. For the time we are on this earth, we have this body to experience. When we connect to our spirit, we connect to the gift it is to be human. This gift includes having a relationship to the outside world, our senses, and our emotions—and perceiving them through a lens of gratitude. Taking pleasure in all that being a human encompasses is a way to show gratitude for the life you have been given. Gratitude is a transcendent emotion, and when applied to all we undergo as humans, it alters our state of consciousness.

Being rooted in this pleasure center shields you from negativity. When you are connected to your pleasure and integrate it with your values, a sense of confidence and worthiness of that pleasure prevents you from feeding into the antagonistic attitudes of those around you; you are too focused on what is true for you. Aligning yourself with this sense of worthiness by fostering a healthy relationship with sexuality affects other areas of your life, too. You become cognizant of the benefits of releasing guilt associated with feeling good.

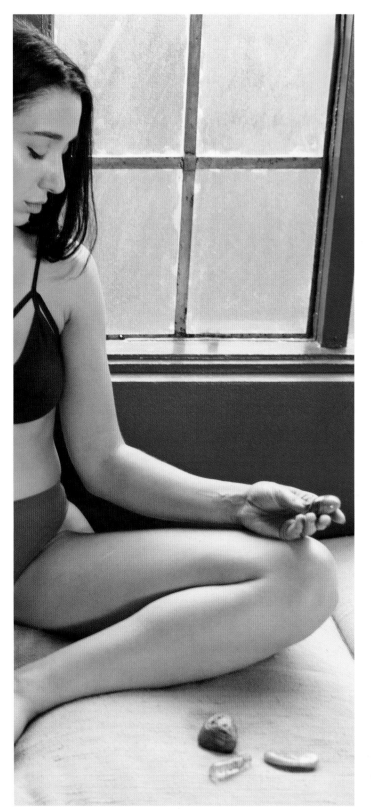

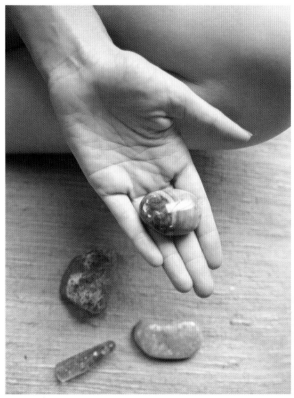

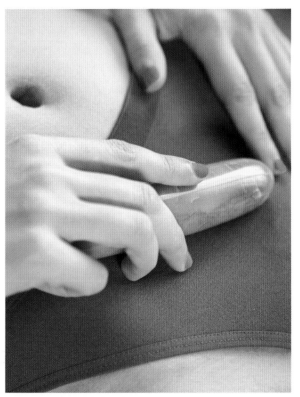

The Gift of Nature:
SACRAL CHAKRA EXERCISE

Because this center focuses on being in tune with subtle pleasures and taking deep joy in them, this exercise will focus on light clitoral stimulation.

The clitoris is the only organ on the body that's only purpose is pleasure. As such, it is the perfect place for honoring the sacral chakra—the chakra dedicated specifically to the pleasurable aspects of sexuality. The clitoris, like every other part of the vulva, is different on every body. Most people think of it as the little hooded part at the top of the vagina, but it is actually made up of four parts: the clit tip, the prepuce (sometimes referred to as the "clitoral hood"), the body (shaft), and the legs—the full shape is much like that of a wishbone. When not aroused, the clit tip is on average about half a centimeter long. This tiny area is filled with 8,000 nerve endings, and the surrounding areas add even more, which is why the area is so pleasurable to touch.

The full size and scope of the clitoris wasn't discovered until 1998, when urologist Helen O'Connell began studying it using MRI. She was able to prove that much of the clitoris's anatomy—about 4 inches (10 cm) of it—is actually inside the pelvis. When a woman becomes aroused, the clitoral legs swell around the vagina, creating a cuff that is stimulated with pleasure. This information has challenged our understanding of vaginal orgasms, as we now know that orgasms achieved through penetration are often a type of clitoral orgasm.

The word *clitoris* comes from the Greek root word *kleitoris*, which translates to "godly" or "goddess-like." Touching this spot is perfect for increasing the transcendental feeling of gratitude for life by indulging in the joy of this gift of nature.

TIP: You may wish to start with the labia massage explained in the Root Chakra Ritual (page 105) as a warm-up.

Create your space for this exercise. First, make sure your hands are thoroughly cleansed with mild, gentle soap. Because you will be lying flat on your back, create a nesting place on your bed or floor. Keep your Chakrub, yoni egg, or sacral crystal nearby. Start by stating your sacral chakra intention. For example, "I feel connected and love for my body," or simply, "I feel." For this exercise, start completely naked, or undressed from the waist down, if you choose to do the sensual touching aspect of this exercise.

TIP: If you don't have a clitoris or wish to open/heal the sacral chakra, you can place the orange crystal of your choice on the area 4 inches (10 cm) below your navel and perform the non-sensual touching parts of this exercise.

Choose Your Crystals

Crystals for this exercise will ideally be orange or peach in color. A Chakrub or yoni egg is best, though to receive the support of another crystal, you can hold it in your less dominant hand while performing the massage with your dominant hand. Follow the steps below, but make it your own. This practice will last about 15 minutes, but can go as long as you'd like.

1. Sit with the soles of your feet touching (you may wish to sit on a blanket or pillow for added comfort). This is a butterfly pose, which will call in transformative animal energy. Hold your sacral chakra crystal in your less dominant hand and begin to mindfully breathe in through the nose, out through the mouth. You may also sit in a comfortable chair, if you prefer.

2. Tune in to the energy of the crystal. Imagine it is connected to your sacral chakra, the area about 4 inches (10 cm) below your navel. Visualize the crystal residing there, glowing in a beautiful sunset orange.

3. Take note of any changes in sensation you feel. Do you feel heat, coolness, or tingling sensation?

4. Gently lay down on your back, keeping the soles of your feet touching. Continue to breathe.

5. Place your crystal on the sacral chakra area and deepen your breath to meet the crystal in your lower stomach. Continue this breathing.

6. Once you feel ready, move your yoni egg or Chakrub to your dominant hand and touch it lightly to your clitoris. If you do not have a yoni egg or Chakrub, continue to hold the sacral crystal over your sacral chakra with your less dominant hand, and touch the area with your dominant hand. *Optional:* Before making physical contact with this area, grab a mirror and observe it without judgments. If you choose to do this, take your time as if you were "eye-gazing" with this part of yourself.

7. With ever-so-slight pressure (like the wings of a butterfly), touch the area to the right of the clitoris, and see if you can strengthen the sensation by feeling the energy of the crystal.

8. Repeat on the left side of the clitoris. Try moving in circles, strokes, or whatever feels good. Remember to breathe.

9. Be mindful of any sensations you feel. Imagine the energy you created moving up to your sacral chakra. Visualize the orange sunset glow in your chakra glowing brighter and brighter. You may choose to say the sensual sound associated with this chakra, *"oo."*

10. Rest your crystal on your sacral chakra.

11. *Optional:* Because the sacral chakra is associated with sense of taste, you may wish to end this exercise by tasting yourself.

Materials

· Blanket or pillow, optional

· Comfortable chair, optional

· Crystal (see pages 120 through 123)

Extras for the Sacral Chakra

Because the sacral chakra is associated with the sense of taste, mindful indulgence in eating delicious and healthy foods is another way to awaken this center.

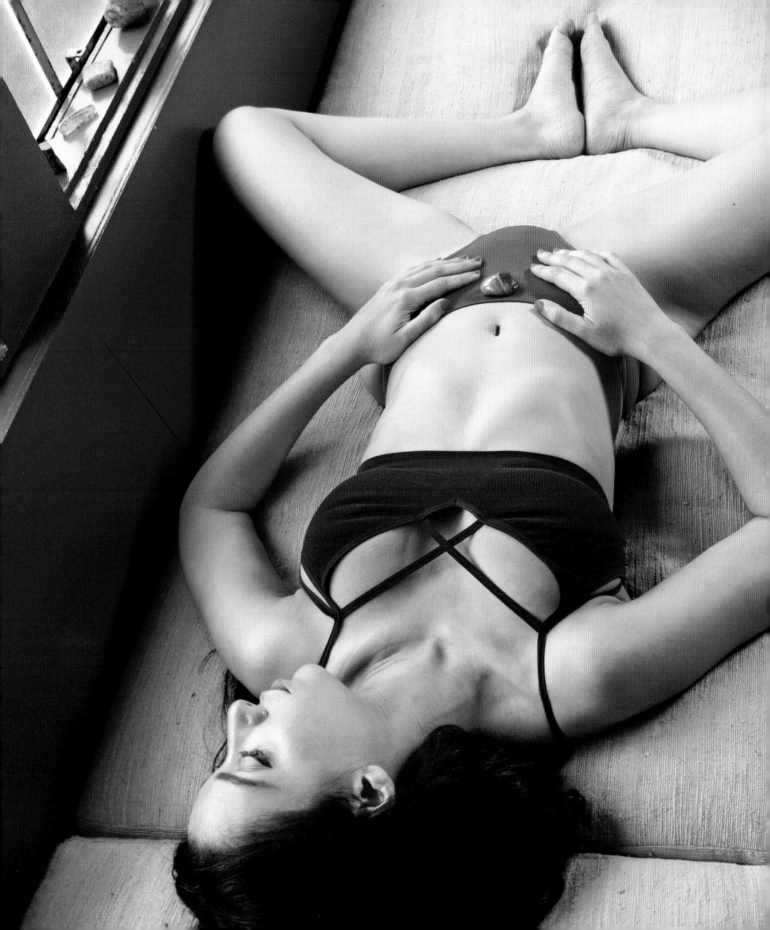

Crystals for the Sacral Chakra

The sacral chakra is associated with the color orange, and because its element is water, it could also take the color of very light blue or white in more rare occasions. Crystals of this color will strengthen this chakra and can be used to strengthen creativity, bring light and levity to serious situations, and strengthen long-term commitments.

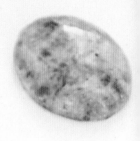

SUNSTONE

ORANGE AVENTURINE

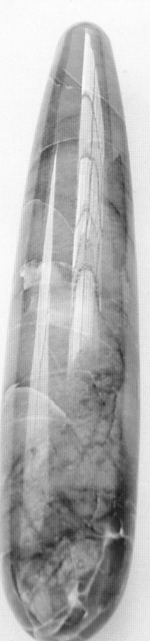

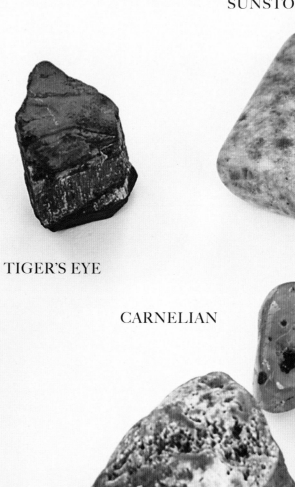

TIGER'S EYE

CARNELIAN

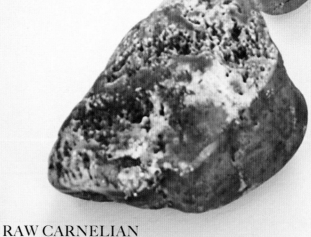

RAW CARNELIAN

CARNELIAN

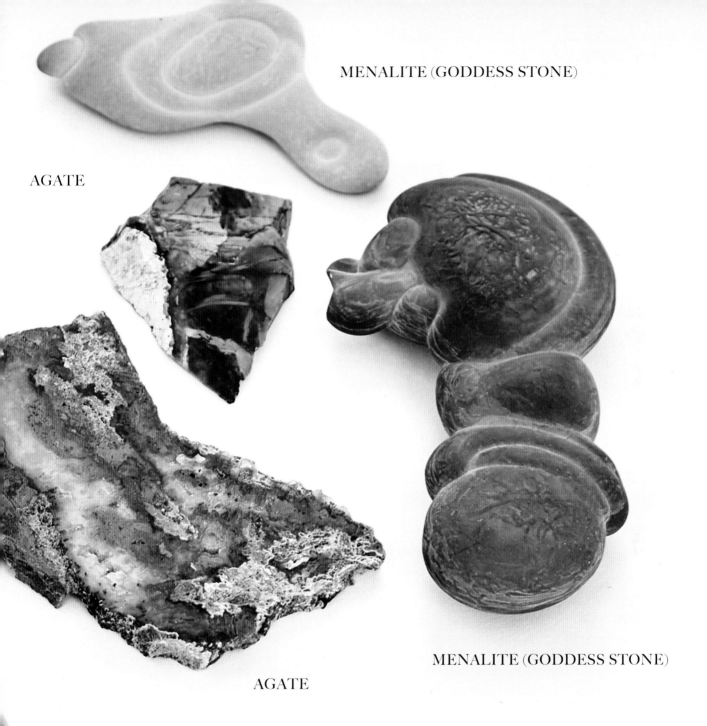

MENALITE (GODDESS STONE)

AGATE

MENALITE (GODDESS STONE)

AGATE

Carnelian

Carnelian is a brilliant, orange or red-colored variety of chalcedony that's name is derived from the Latin word for flesh. Ancient Egyptians associated this stone with the fertile menstrual blood of the mother goddess, Isis. That's fitting, as carnelian is known to stimulate blood flow and influence the reproductive organs of both sexes.

BENEFITS:

Traditionally used to enhance passion, love, and desire

— Known as the "Singer's Stone," it clarifies the voice

— Used for the consummation of love and to rekindle passion

— Restores vitality and stimulates creativity

— Evokes confidence and helps overcome sexual anxieties and eating disorders

— Protects against envy, rage, or resentment from yourself and others

Sunstone

Sunstone is a joyful stone named for its warm shades of red, orange, gold, and brown that sparkle like the sun. It carries the energy of Ra, the sun god, whose radiant energy brings all potential life from within the Earth.

BENEFITS:

Inspires the nurturing self and to be of service to others

— Inspires leadership and personal power

— Reflecting the qualities of light, stimulates openness, warmth, and generosity

— Provides strength to those dealing with loss or emotional dependence

— Vitalizes and energizes while stimulating self-healing powers

— Removes hooks from possessive loved ones or lovers

— Helps strengthen resolve for those who have difficulty saying no

— Can acts as an antidepressant for those with seasonal affective disorder

Orange Aventurine

Orange aventurine is sometimes called the "Whisper Stone" because it can quiet a critical inner voice and promote self-love. It is a powerful stone of good fortune and helps align its wearer with their highest vibration.

BENEFITS:

Promotes feelings of calm and balance

— Stills the mind during meditation

— Helpful for dealing with issues of self-worth and increasing confidence

— Promotes creative problem solving to overcome challenges

— Promotes clear communication and enhances intellectualism

— Manifests new opportunities and encourages ideas

— Helps with healing from sexual trauma

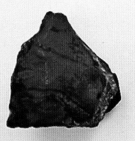

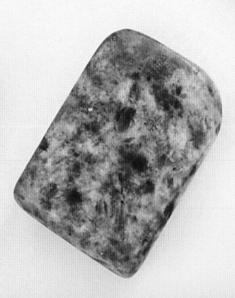

Tiger's Eye

Tiger's Eye is a balancing stone that synthesizes the energy frequencies of the sun and earth. An ancient talisman revered by many cultures, tiger's eye has been called the "all-seeing and all-knowing eye" for its ability to give its wearer greater insight and observational skills. Egyptians gave their deity statues eyes made with tiger's eye to symbolize divine wisdom.

BENEFITS:

Invokes compassion and practicality in decision-making

— Wards off complacency and stimulates an open mind eager to try new things

— Helps piece together fragmented information

— Inspires creativity and utilizing one's talents

— Sharpens vision and provides a bird's-eye view of situations

— Stimulates personal will to help break bad habits or addictions

— Sparks imagination and intuition and can assist in dream recollection

Menalite
(goddess or fairy stone)

Menalite occurs naturally by forming in Quaternary deposits left in lakes by receding glaciers. Native Americans have referred to them as "fairy stones" for centuries and carried them for good luck and protection against negative entities. Today we call menalite the goddess stone, as it enhances our connection with the divine feminine. Its formations are unusual and often recall animals and goddess-like carvings.

BENEFITS:

Boosts intuition and creative and manifestation powers

— Creates a connection to wise feminine and goddess energy

— Can be used for shamanic journeying and astral travel

— Balances masculine and feminine energies

— Restores connection to the earth and grounds energy

— Calls forth the energies needed to realize one's purpose in this lifetime

— Emphasizes the naturally occurring life cycles of rebirth and reincarnation

— Provides support when dealing with loss or death

— Supports fertility, menopause, menstruation, and lactation

Agate

Referred to as the "earth rainbow" for its beautiful banded layers and stripes, agate has been used for healing dating back to the times of Babylon. Some agates have markings that appears like eyes. Throughout history there are reports of agate revealing divine figures in its natural veining, such as the Virgin Mary, Jesus, John the Baptist, and angels. These natural works of art are still celebrated in various churches and museums throughout the world today.

BENEFITS:

Vibrates at a lower frequency that contains a stabilizing and strengthening influence

— Harmonizes yin and yang and balances emotional energy

— Removes desire for things we don't need

— Can be used as a support crystal during pregnancy and postpartum to avoid depression

— Promotes fidelity within committed relationships

— Encourages realistic and pragmatic thinking

— Helps one overcome bitterness and negativity by healing anger and fostering love

— Useful for overcoming trauma

— Helpful in identifying circumstances that are detrimental to one's well-being

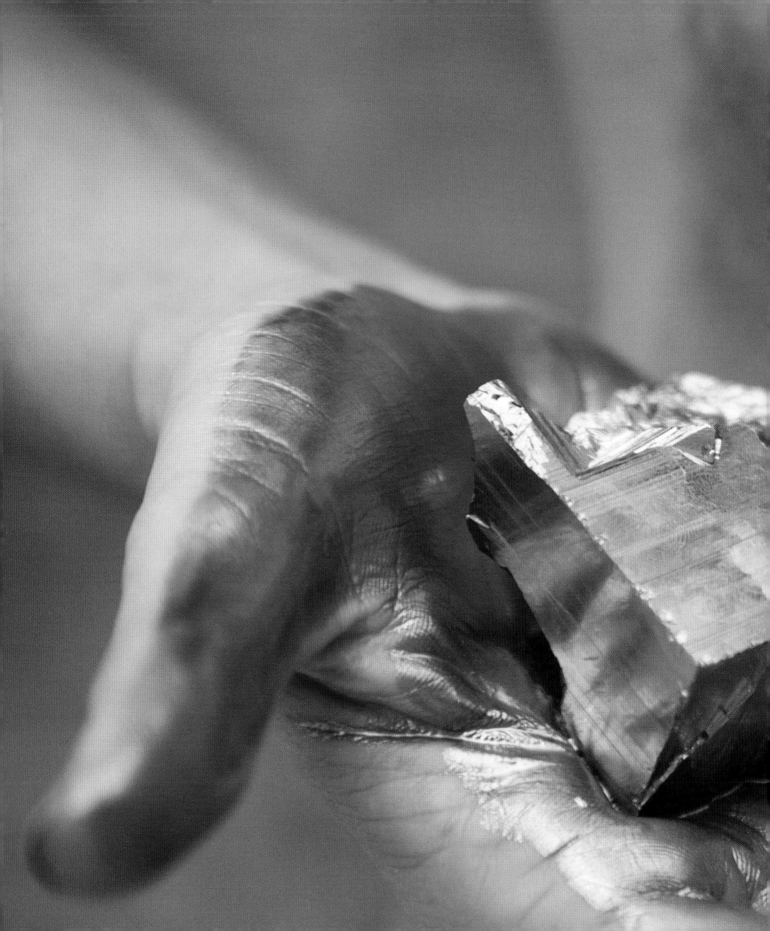

8 | THE SOLAR PLEXUS CHAKRA

The solar plexus is in the navel. When we have a "gut" feeling, we are tuning in to the wisdom of this energy center. It manages our digestion, not just of food but also as we process our thoughts in accordance with our will. It is here that we learn to culminate our sexual energy to manifest desires in the physical realm.

According to Buddhist theory, the solar plexus chakra, also called *Manipura*, is the seat of Kundalini energy. The first two chakras, the root chakra and the sacral chakra, represent higher ranges of primal life, while human consciousness begins at Manipura and becomes refined as Kundalini energy moves upward. It is a pale yellow to deep gold color. It is associated with the pancreas, which aides in digestion and helps regulate blood sugar, and the solar plexus, a bunch of nerves branching from the abdominal aorta. When you feel stressed or anxious, you'll feel the solar plexus as a tight knot below the sternum or a hollow feeling in your stomach. This chakra manages the digestive system, skin, diaphragm, small intestines, and upper abdomen.

The energetic archetype of this chakra is the Warrior. It provides the belly of courage to go forth on a worthy path. Spending time focusing on this chakra awakens joy for sexuality, giving the overall expression and understanding of it a sense of lightheartedness. It is here we remember to not take ourselves too seriously and, in this way, we activate our personal power, one which is not overruled by our ego.

A Healthy Solar Plexus Chakra

When the solar plexus chakra is functioning well, you are tuned in to your personal power. You have clear ideas of your values, and you can prioritize your responses to situations based on those values, so you feel successful. Because you're rooted in success based on your personal values, you can take responsibility for your life and not put unfair pressure on others to create your happiness. You understand the power you have in the creation of your life as a whole and in daily situations. You feel confident asking for what you desire sexually or emotionally, and you ask for it directly without being domineering. When this energy center is balanced, you practice healthy assertiveness and find ease in cooperation.

In relationships, someone with a balanced and healthy solar plexus chakra is willing to take risks. You are fearless due to the power of the confidence and self-assurance that are accessed here. You find patience and joy in relationships, because you know they can be positively created through trust with gut emotions.

When the Solar Plexus Chakra Needs Acknowledgment

When the solar plexus chakra is functioning poorly, you can easily become emotionally manipulated or turn to emotional manipulation to get what you want from others. You may fall into victimhood, and you may even create issues to receive attention. This shows a need for power but the disbelief that you have it. A person with a poorly functioning solar plexus chakra could enter servitude, serving others while neglecting the self, with the secret hope of receiving recognition or creating dependency in the person being served.

Solar Plexus Chakra Snapshot

Color: Yellow

Sensual Sound: *Oh*

Musical Tone: E

Location: Slightly to the left above the stomach

Governs: Sense of personal power, fulfillment

Healthy: Confidence, willpower

Unhealthy: Nervousness, digestive issues

Sense: Sight

Organ: Eyes

Sexuality: Joyous union

Element: Fire

Intention: I Do

Word Origin: Solar Plexus Chakra

The Sanskrit word for the third chakra is *Manipura*, which translates to "city of gems." This imagery comes into play because the solar plexus chakra is responsible for our self-esteem, sense of purpose, and personal identity—all the gems we bestow on the world.

When this chakra is deficient, a person may experience low self-esteem and look to engage in sex acts to create a fleeting sense of power or significance. It can also manifest as a lack of self-confidence resulting in self-sabotage. Because of a lack of self-confidence and a belief that their actions do not really matter, a person with deficiencies in this chakra could be passive and seen as unreliable, due to not valuing their own significance in a situation. Self-judgment and criticism can also drain the energy of this chakra and will weaken personal willpower.

When the third chakra is excessive, a person may be domineering and have an imbalanced understanding of their power in a situation through means of aggression and control. Blaming others, hostility, and mean-spirited language signify an excess in this chakra.

Learning to Laugh

A healthy solar plexus results in ease of humor, one of my favorite erotic arts. Laughter, whether we are causing it or experiencing it, is incredibly sexy.

It took me quite some time, as well as support from the right partner, to learn to laugh. I lost my virginity to a man six years older than me; the first time we had sex, I was far from ready to enter into my sexuality. Not wanting to accept my first time as a negative experience, I decided to foster a relationship with him. But my pleasure was not a priority in our relationship, and I did not know enough about sexuality to tell him what I needed. I was thoroughly disappointed in sex, as I'd always thought it would be profound and feel amazing. I relinquished this idea and bought into the idea that sex was mainly for him. I learned how to make it look and feel especially good for him so he would finish quickly, so that I could relax. I disassociated from my body. I did this for six years.

After the relationship ended, I created the idea for Chakrubs: I finally took pleasure into my own hands, creating something that would not only help me to achieve the deepest orgasms of my life but help respond to my emotional wounds. It was only after I began employing crystals to put pleasure back in my body that I realized that who and what I allow to enter me should be energetically ordained, with the purpose to make me feel good.

It wasn't until my current relationship that I could incorporate these ideas into my sex life with a partner. My partner has taught me through his own ability to remain authentic, that sex doesn't always have to be some intense, lavish, porn-worthy endeavor. It can be relaxed, it can take time, and it can hold humor. Laughing together during sex helps us to relieve pressure of performance, to just "be," to remove the stress of orgasm from every sexual encounter, and take to pleasure in simplicity. After all, we are most powerful when we remove tension from our bodies and minds.

You Are Sacred Space:
SOLAR PLEXUS CHAKRA RITUAL

For this exercise, you will be honoring your body as a sacred space for manifesting that which you desire in the outside world. Whether it be a promotion, adventures through travel, or a new home, this practice elevates your energy to be a vibrational match for obtaining it. First, honor the courage you have for acknowledging your desires and acting upon them. Then, honor your body as a powerful force of energy that you can ignite to create what you want. Because this chakra is about manifesting what we desire on the material realm, we use a crystal grid. Here we affirm how our body is sacred space by employing it as the foundation.

A crystal grid is created by placing crystals in a pattern to generate energy toward a specific intention. Grids can be used in connection with sacred geometry—patterns that hold spiritual significance. You can draw or print these patterns and overlay your crystals on them, or use your intuition and creativity to arrange your crystals in a way that feels good to you. The way the crystals are arranged helps concentrate external energies into a single, powerful forcefield tuned to a specific intention. This unified energy field creates a flow of vibrational interactions between the crystals' energies and the aura, mind, and spirit of the person conducting the grid. This should be a fun and creative process.

Choose a space to perform this ritual. You will be laying down flat on your back, preferably on a yoga mat on a flat surface. You could do this outside in the sun for added energy.

Stonehenge: A Crystal Grid

Stonehenge in Wiltshire, England, is an example of a large grid that may have been created to amplify prayers in that area. Constructed over a span of at least 1,500 years, it is one of the most famous prehistoric sites in the world. It was constructed to perfectly align with the two solstices, and is at one of only two latitudes in the world where the full moon passes directly overhead during its maximum altitudes. Some suspect that to people of its time, Stonehenge represented the center of the world.

Crystal grids employ multiple crystals, so you will be creating your own "city of gems" dedicated to your intention. Placing crystals around your home and connecting them with a wand is another way to employ this practice. Start by placing crystals around your home or room. Take a crystal wand and hold it toward each crystal. As you walk toward the next crystal, hold the wand toward your heart.

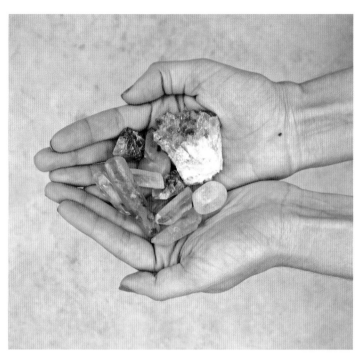

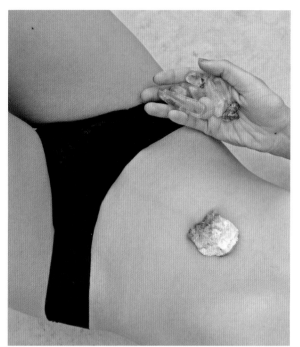

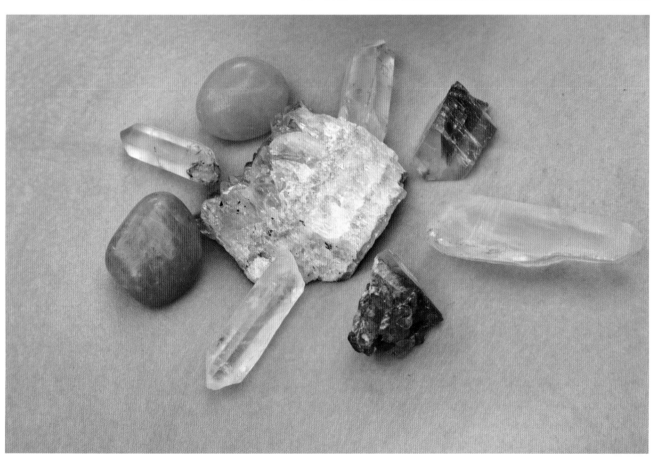

Choose Your Crystals

You can use any crystals that you have. Typically, grids use a master stone in the center as a focal point and generator, as well as a wand to connect the surrounding crystals to the master. Here are the components of a crystal grid:

- **Master or focus stone:** This stone is usually the largest in the grid. It gathers and focuses the intention and universal life force energy.

- **Way stones:** These are the stones immediately surrounding the focus stone. The focus stone pulls down universal life force energy, and the way stones direct the energy outward.

- **Desire stones:** These stones are on the outermost area of the grid. They represent the intention that you desire.

- **The path:** The path is the invisible lines of energy connecting all the components of the crystal grid. It represents the flow of energy in the grid.

- **The wand:** The wand crystal is what is used to activate the energy of the grid and direct energy flow for each crystal.

Gather your crystals for this ritual. Choose one master stone (typically the largest) and one wand. This exercise takes 15 minutes.

1. State your intention. Because this chapter focuses on the solar plexus, your intention can be to manifest what you desire in any area of your life. If you aren't sure, it can simply be, "I create that which I desire with ease." If you have a something specific you want to manifest, you may choose to write it down on a piece of paper.

2. Place your crystals nearby and lay down on a yoga mat. Tune in to your breath, and when you feel ready, clearly state your intention.

3. Place your master crystal directly on your solar plexus chakra, about 2 inches (5 cm) above the belly button.

4. Place your way stones and your desire stones. You can add or subtract as many crystals as you want. You may wish to keep them close to the center of your belly so they don't fall over. Call on your intuition to place them in the grid.

5. Take the wand in your dominant hand and point it toward the master stone. State your intention and tune in to the energy of the crystals.

6. Energetically connect the crystals to the master stone by pointing the wand to each crystal surrounding it and then bringing it back to the master stone.

7. Once all the crystals are connected, relax and continue to breathe.

Materials

- Piece of paper and pen, optional
- Crystals (see pages 134 through 137)
- Yoga mat

Extras for the Solar Plexus Chakra

Because the solar plexus chakra is associated with the sense of sight, creating a vision board can be useful in strengthening this area. A vision board is a display of images that help you to envision that which you desire. You can print out or cut out images from magazines that represent the things you want or draw them yourself.

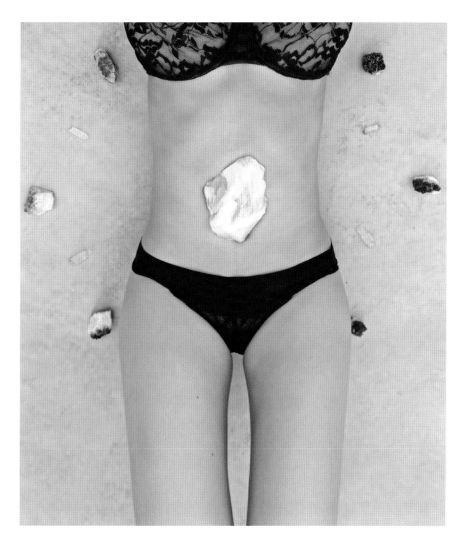

Alternate Crystal Grid:

1. Follow the steps on the previous page, this time by placing the way stones and desire stones around the area where you will be laying down.

2. Keep the master stone on your solar plexus chakra. You are the center of this grid.

3. Connect each crystal as you would in the previous exercise.

4. *Optional*: Employ the orgasmic manifestation method described on the next page.

Orgasmic Manifestation

The mind becomes so clear at the moment of orgasm that the experience has been likened to death, or as the French call it, *le petit mort*. The ego is suspended as we enter into a state of complete surrender. Orgasmic energy brings our vibration to its highest state, free of identity and open to receiving. We can employ this heightened state to match the energy of that which we want in our lives. This is called Orgasmic Manifestation, or Sex Magic. We crave orgasms for a sense of relief and to bring forth new energy into our world.

Think about the word *conception*. When we refer to the date we were conceived, we trace back to the moment our parents joined in union to create a human life. Conception and orgasm are creative forces. Whatever you are focusing or feeling in the moments leading up to an orgasm will be conceived.

There are two main types of orgasm: explosive and implosive. An explosive orgasm happens when the energy moves out of the body. It is most natural for male-bodied people and is ideal for releasing stress and for manifestation work. An implosive orgasm occurs when you draw your partner's (or your crystal's) energy into yours. This is the best kind of orgasm for healing or unity and comes most naturally to female-bodied people. Where an explosive orgasm can leave you depleted, an implosive orgasm expands within you to restore your energy. One of the drawbacks of an implosive orgasm is that it can become a crutch for those who fear surrendering themselves during sex and can lead to excessive amounts of energy. Both types of orgasms have their benefits, so it is wise to be mindful about what kind of orgasm serves your current needs and desires.

The solar plexus chakra is all about being connected to personal power, and manifesting through the power of orgasmic energy does just that. When I first began my self-healing process, I changed the process by which I became aroused. Instead of thinking about common fantasies to get aroused, I would imagine what it would feel like if I were to be making love to someone I loved. This led me to clearly understand what I wanted: to hear and say "I love you" during sex. I could then embody the energy of the kind of partner I wanted to manifest. This was my first introduction to manifesting through orgasm, but it doesn't stop at manifesting love.

If you already have a specific idea of what you want to invoke more of in your life, you can channel your own orgasmic energy into receiving it. There are two ways to practice this. One, as I mentioned earlier, is to embody the energy you call in while you are in a heightened state of sensual pleasure and attract what you want into your life. The second method is to develop a clear focus on what you want to manifest, with a strong visual component or intention. Hold it in your mind. At the moment of orgasm, state your intention aloud or focus on your visual. With practice, this will be a powerful tool. As you approach orgasm, energy builds up, waiting to be released. This can be done with a partner or alone. If you and your partner have a shared intention, all the better!

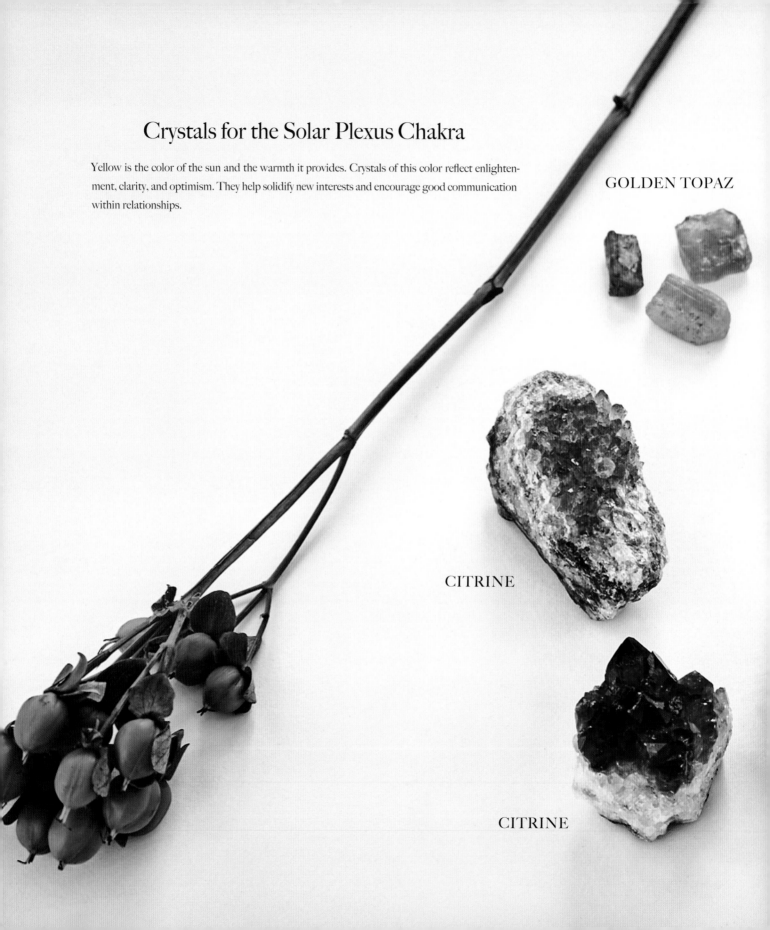

Crystals for the Solar Plexus Chakra

Yellow is the color of the sun and the warmth it provides. Crystals of this color reflect enlightenment, clarity, and optimism. They help solidify new interests and encourage good communication within relationships.

GOLDEN TOPAZ

CITRINE

CITRINE

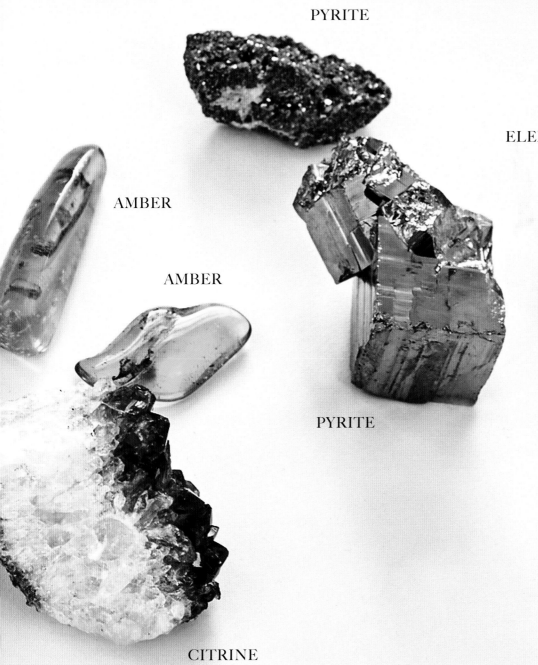

PYRITE

ELEMENTAL SULFUR

AMBER

AMBER

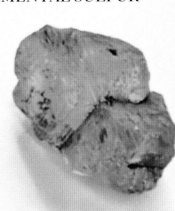

PYRITE

CITRINE

Citrine

A transparent, yellow variety of quartz, citrine carries the power of the sun and invigorates its wearer by inspiring creativity and authentic self-expression. It is thought to detoxify the circulatory system and is associated in many ancient cultures with blood and life-force energy. Citrine is useful for dissipating, transmuting, and grounding energies and is one of two stones that does not need to be cleansed.

BENEFITS:

Ideal for inviting in manifestation and abundance

— Assists in releasing negativity from the past and assimilating lessons

— Raises self-esteem and promotes an optimistic outlook

— Purifies personal will for the greatest good

— Assists in identifying and healing issues of power abuse and helplessness

— Promotes cohesion in interpersonal relationships

— Guards against those who will break your heart

— Shields against spite and jealousy

— Enhances physical stamina

Amber

Known as the "Gold of the Sea," amber is intrinsically formed by light and life and preserved by time in a protective resin that oozed from living trees in dense, prehistoric forests and fossilized over millions of years. It has been used as a talisman for beauty, protection, and renewal since the Stone Age.

BENEFITS:

Transmutes negative or stagnant energies into positive, light energy

— Ideal for battling addictions, suicidal thoughts, depression, anxiety, and seasonal affective disorder

— Stimulates the body's ability to heal itself

— Assists in removing obstacles created by the self and deflects negative energies

— Lends courage to set boundaries and recognize personal power in a loving way

— Enhances understanding of past events to aid in present decision-making and forward movement

— Helps align the personality with the spiritual self

— Protects from psychic attacks

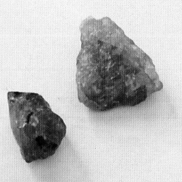

Pyrite

Pyrite is called "Fool's Gold" because of its visual similarity to gold. The name comes from the Greek word *Pyr*, which means fire. It was given this name for its ability to create the sparks needed to start a fire.

BENEFITS:

Protects against negative energies and environmental pollution

— Promotes physical health and well-being

— Attracts abundance, wealth, and prosperity

— Encourages one to take confident action

— Guards against manipulation by a partner, parent, or employer and changes the balance of power

— Enhances protective and assertive masculine energies

— Increases self-worth and helps women overcome tendencies toward servitude and inferiority

— For men, instills confidence in one's masculinity and promotes healthy expression of sexuality

— Promotes positive thoughts and helps overcome misfortune or despair

— Can be used to create harmony within the auric field

Golden Topaz

This stone carries a strong healing vibration that will aid in manifestation and is an excellent tool for connecting with the divine. Keeping this stone within your auric fields will ease stress and irritability.

BENEFITS:

Harnesses the energy of the sun to promote vibrancy, generosity, and strength

— Promotes clarity when creating intentions and taps into inner resources

— Brings awareness of personal influence and helps transform life experiences into lessons

— Recharges the spirit as well as the physical body and strengthens faith and optimism

— Promotes healthiness and clears up disorders in the body

— Promotes emotional stability

— Amplifies connection to angelic realms

Elemental Sulfur

Volcanic in origin, sulfur is a purifying crystal that absorbs negativity and helps connect with one's higher purpose. It vitalizes by allowing its user to perceive situations in new ways. Caution: When combined with other elements and stones, sulfur can be toxic. Take care in handling this stone and do not place it in water.

BENEFITS:

Increases focus

— Aids in solidifying new interests and relationships

— A helpful tool for those seeking enlightenment

— Encourages a healthy optimism and gives meaning to life and relationships

— Allows one to release negativity in a productive manner

— Encourages one to be flexible and go with the flow

— Helps release negative patterns that are blocking abundance

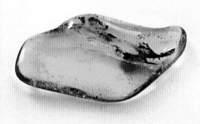
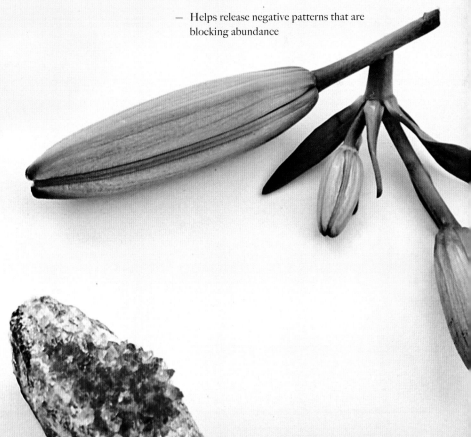

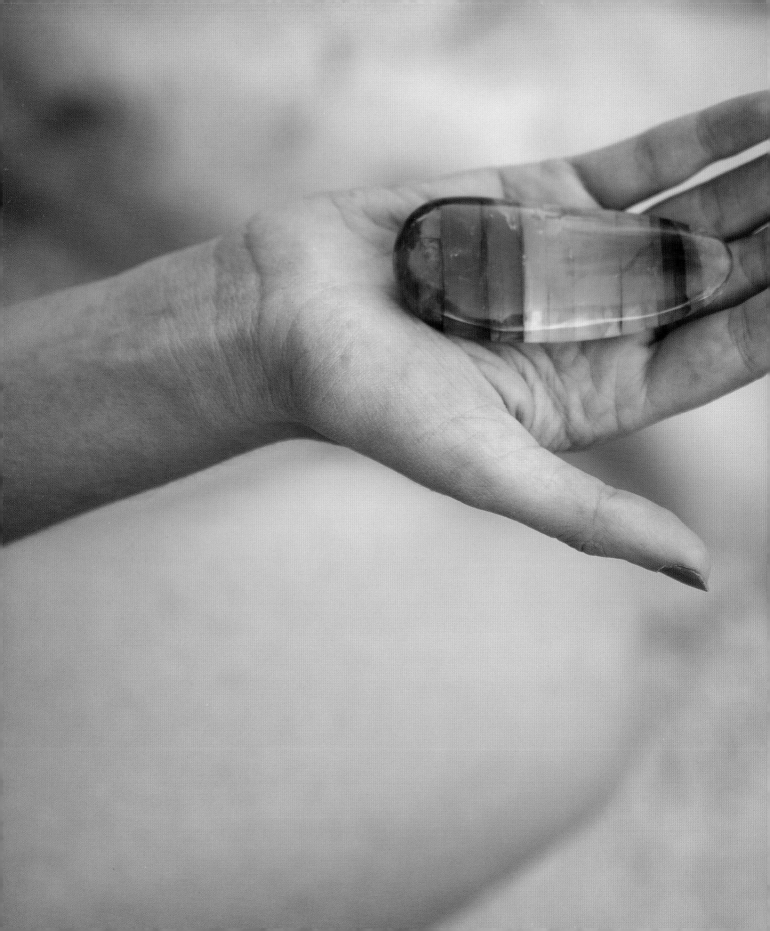

9 | THE HEART CHAKRA

The heart chakra is at the center of the chest. It is also at the center of the seven main chakras, connecting our relationship between our earthly and physical awareness to our understanding of more spiritual levels. Learning to tune in to the heart center and allow it to remain open gives you a sense of peace as well as the ability to connect with goodness, regardless of circumstance. When this chakra is healthy, the heart beats in perfect rhythm, creating our internal music.

Ancient Taoists referred to the breasts as "bells of love," and it is believed that the breasts are gateways to the heart center. For male-bodied people or people who do not have breasts (due to mastectomies, for example) there are still energetic breasts to be felt from within.

Because this chakra lies at our heart center, it helps support our cardiac system and lungs. It manages the heart, circulatory system, cardiac plexus, thymus gland, lungs, breasts, and the lymphatic system. It's responsible for hormone production and helps regulate the immune system.

Regarded as the most significant nerve in the parasympathetic nervous system, the vagus nerve travels throughout the body and is responsible for the mind-body connection. It has different functions depending on where in the body it is, but plays an important role in gut and brain health. It promotes digestion in the belly, regulates the heart rate and blood pressure, and helps control fertility and orgasm in women. You can activate the vagus nerve through the heart chakra by making a deep "Ah" sound. This will cause the vagus nerve to vibrate, sending signals to relax.

The energy archetype of this chakra is The Lover. The heart chakra is how we regulate our relationships, ensuring that we give love to ourselves as much as we give love to others, as well as to The Divine.

A Healthy Heart Chakra

When in balance, the heart chakra connects us to calm emotions and an overall feeling of peace. Through acceptance and empathy, we can see the beauty in all there is. This doesn't mean that we have to like everything but our boundaries are set with love and we act with assertiveness rather than aggression, bringing forth an air of love. Working on the heart chakra alone can have tremendous effects on all the chakras.

Love is a state of being not reliant on circumstances. When this chakra is nurtured and functioning clearly, we can experience love in many capacities. We can see past judgments of ourselves or others and bring peace to many situations. Our love is not based on the object being loved; it is our disposition. It is through healing and vitalizing the heart center that one understands that by loving others, you love yourself. Every relationship, be it with an acquaintance or family member or intimate partner, is a reflection of your relationship with yourself. Love is in part intuition and feeling, and it's in part a decision. This is, again, the bridge between the higher chakras and lower chakras.

Some of us may fear cultivating a strong relationship to the self, but doing it will increase our capability for loving others. It's not true that there are "no good men" or "no good women" anymore. The true issue is that we all need to develop ourselves so that we can see to the depths of the people around us and recognize them for the gods and goddesses they are.

Heart Chakra Snapshot

Color: Pale green through vibrant emerald to deep forest green

Secondary Color: Pink

Sensual Sound: *Ah*

Musical Tone: F

Location: Between the breasts

Governs: Connection between emotional and physical love

Healthy: Compassionate, empathetic, able to surrender to sexual bliss, unconditional love

Unhealthy: Conditional love, possessive, controlling

Sense: Touch

Organ: Skin

Sexuality: Love

Element: Air

Intention: I Love

When the Heart Chakra Needs Acknowledgment

Word Origin: Heart Chakra

The Sanskrit word for the heart chakra is *Anahata*, which translates to "unstuck sound."

Because of the heart's concern with unconditional love, it is here that we also explore that which opposes unconditional love—jealousy, false judgment, and apathy. When this chakra is deficient, forgiveness can be quite difficult. We may hold on to resentment in relationships, romantic or otherwise. This could lead to the desire to punish or seek revenge against anyone we deem to have betrayed us. We can look at our partners and friends with contempt. Lack of empathy lends itself to holding on to grief for ideas of what "should have" been. Issues with self-love arise due to becoming overwhelmed by loneliness—not acknowledging the well of love that is ever-present within. When this chakra has excess energies, it leads to jealousy, a call-to-action emotion. Without listening to the heart, it becomes difficult to make choices that are in alignment with our soul's path, and we become concerned with the desires of more shallow realms.

The Heart Center's Role in Shadow Work

It is here that we find love for ourselves, understanding that our chakra imbalances and the actions we've made because of them are part of our journey. There is no reason to feel ashamed. Imposing a compassionate understanding of ourselves—even in our "deficient" areas—is critical to this work. The heart center is home to all positive virtues. Without this connection to the heart, we would not be able to experience the blessings of shadow work—confronting the parts of ourselves that we've previously decided are shameful. We're able to meet ourselves, our perversions, our lust, our anxiety, or our defiance through a compassionate lens. Making peace with them allows us to make peace with their presence in the world, furthering our connection to all. We do not necessarily have to like that these things are present, but we understand their place as part of the divine universe. We give honor to ourselves, and we honor the universe.

The Bells of the Heart:
HEART CHAKRA EXERCISE

You can satisfy your need for nourishment by giving attention to your breasts. Massaging them reminds us that when we take care of ourselves first, we are better suited to care for others. Playing with our breasts nurtures our inner child.

When aroused, the breasts swell up to 25 percent. There are even women who have reported breast growth due to regular breast massage. Where attention goes, energy flows. Thinking of the breasts as an extension of the heart chakra, it is truly amazing to see how imbuing love into this area causes physical growth.

To begin this exercise, find a quiet place where you will not be interrupted for about one hour. Dress the area with items or pleasant aromas that bring you a sense of comfort. Clean your hands and undress the upper part of your body. Place your heart chakra crystal massager and optional massage oil nearby.

TIP: If you don't have breasts or nipples, you can do this exercise energetically by focusing your attention to the field of energy 1 to 2 inches (2.5 to 5 cm) away from the chest, or massage the areas of the chest that feel right for you.

The Benefits of Breast Massage

Massage is a reliable way to drain the breasts' lymphatic system and create a path for nutrient-rich blood to travel to the breast tissue. Recent science indicates that breast massage is a healthy way to fight cancer, but this practice has been alive and well for thousands of years. Environmental toxins are stored in fatty breast tissue. These harmful toxins can impede healthy circulation in the breasts, and too much toxic buildup can increase your chance of developing breast cancer in the future. Regular breast massage allows our bodies to clear those toxins. And simply familiarizing yourself with the look and shape of your breasts could help you detect any abnormalities in the future.

Along with clearing toxins, breasts release hormones when they're massaged. These hormones include oxytocin, which is called "the love hormone" and has been proven to decrease stress and depression; prolactin, which has been shown to increase breast size when released through massage; and estrogen, which along with all of these hormones, is known to have anti-aging qualities. Breast massage can also be highly arousing and can increase nipple and breast sensitivity. It can be done alone or with a partner.

Simply knead and stroke the breasts, using mild to moderate pressure, while gently lifting and compressing the tissue. Stimulate the nipples as you're working your way around the breasts, as this will encourage blood flood and increase the production of hormones. This allows new pathways for sensitivity in your brain, and through regular practice you may even be able to orgasm from caressing your breasts and nipples. Breast massage can be done to relieve aching breasts and is particularly useful for soothing the pain associated with breast scarring. It eases soreness in the breast tissue and relaxes tension in the ligaments while reducing pain and swelling. Including crystals in breast massage gives you the added benefit of imbuing the breasts with the metaphysical properties of the crystal that seep into the heart chakra.

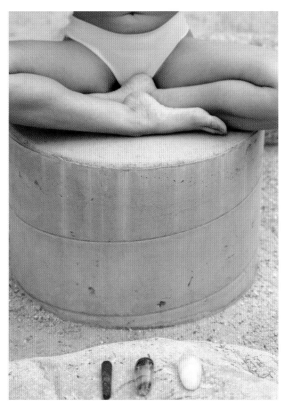

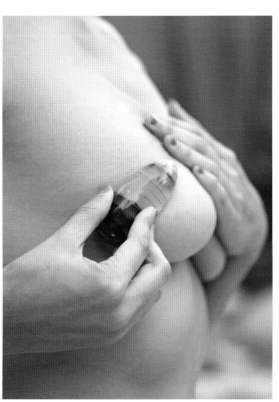

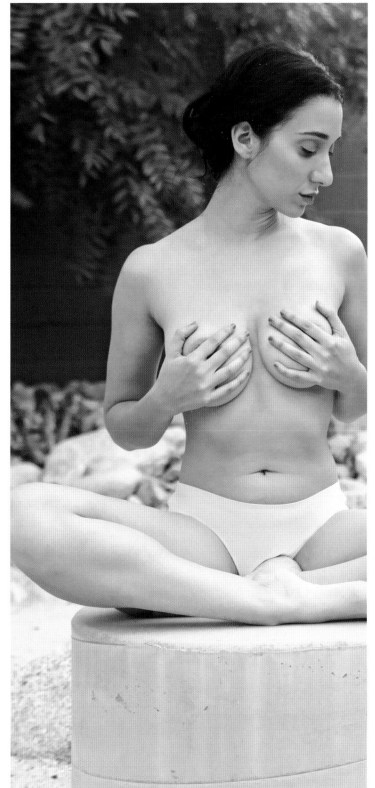

Choose Your Crystals

For this exercise, you will be using your hands or a crystal breast massager. You may prefer to use one that is significant for the heart chakra, but any type will be fine.

Breast crystals are about the length of your palm and have a slight curve to them. If you don't have a breast crystal, you can use a tumbled crystal or one that is completely polished for a smooth surface. You may also choose to use a silk cloth, or even a rose or another flower to perform a soft massage. This practice will take 10 to 15 minutes, or longer if you choose.

Materials

- Cushion, optional
- Rolled towel, optional
- Crystal (see pages 146 through 149)
- Skin-safe massage oil, optional

1. Sit on the floor or comfortably in a chair with your feet on the floor. If sitting on the floor, you can use a cushion to elevate your butt slightly. Place the heel of your foot so it puts gentle pressure on your clitoris, or use a rolled towel to create this pressure. If this is uncomfortable, sitting with your feet on the ground is fine.

2. Set your intention for this practice. Because this is a heart chakra exercise, your intention may be simply, "I love" or "I feel love." Or you may use something more specific that feels good to you.

3. Hold the crystal with your less-dominant hand, with your dominant hand supporting it.

    Breathe deeply while you connect to the crystal. Hold it over your heart chakra in the center of your chest, and allow your heart and the crystal to connect their energies.

4. Place the crystal a comfortable distance in front of you so you can reach it later.

5. Deepen your breathing, and give yourself permission to relax in this time and space. Assure yourself that you are creating healing energy in your body, and smile in gratitude for yourself.

6. Rub your hands together, creating warmth between them. Take a deep breath in and cup your breasts. Wiggle them around, smile, and laugh! This is bringing joy into your breasts and encouraging the flow of stagnant energy. Feel playful, and connect to your inner child. Do this for as long as you need to evoke lightheartedness into this exercise. Feel free to use massage oil for added pleasure.

7. Take a breast in each hand and knead it with a pressure that is comfortable for you, making sure to cover the entire surface area. Say aloud the heart chakra sensual sound, *"ah,"* and visualize your heart chakra opening and spinning as a beautiful green or pink color.

8. While kneading your breasts, you can massage in an outward circle to disperse energy or in an inward circle to gather energy.

9. In Chinese medicine, there is an acupressure point called the Ru Gen point, which is referred to as the "Breast Root Point." It is located directly below the nipples, between your fifth and sixth ribs. Place three fingers on each of your nipples and move them directly down to the bottoms of your breasts. Move them in 2-inch-diameter circles to massage this pressure point.

10. Pick up your breast crystal, and starting with one breast, lightly press the crystal to your nipple and move it in gradually expanding circles until you reach the edges. Repeat on your other breast.

11. Hold the crystal with both hands and feel the energy radiating from your heart into your chest.

12. You can finish this practice by laying down with your crystal resting on your heart, visualizing the healing green color permeating through.

Alternate Heart Chakra Ritual

1. Lay comfortably on your back with your knees propped up on a pillow and your heart chakra crystal nearby.

2. Take your crystal with both hands and rest it in your lap.

3. State your intention to heal, open, and enrich your heart chakra.

4. Place the crystal on your heart center, covering it with your less dominant hand first, then your dominant hand over that.

5. Breathe into the crystal and visualize it within your heart center, radiating its light through your entire body. Do this for approximately five minutes.

6. Rest your hands by your side, allowing the crystal to rest on your heart center.

7. Do this for as long as you'd like, repeating your intentions and visualizing the crystal's color being radiated deep into your heart and throughout your body.

8. When you feel satisfied with this exercise, tap the crystal. Hold it between your hands and thank it and yourself for the work you've done.

Crystals for the Heart Chakra

Crystals in green and pink shades will resonate with the heart chakra. Green crystal energy will help resolve blockages and can restore balance to the heart region. It helps us understand our needs and emotions with more clarity and accept the changes that come in relationships. Pink crystals enhance sensuality and attract new love, romance, and relationships. They offer healing energy to help us overcome heartache and increase our capacity to love.

Rhodonite

First discovered in the rural mountains of Russia, rhodonite was known as the "Eagle Stone" because eagles in the region would gather small pieces for their nests. People in the region began a similar tradition of keeping a piece in babies' cribs. Rhodonite can bring emotional balance after a major loss, heartache, illness, financial disappointment, or period of depression.

BENEFITS:

Encourages one to reclaim their true purpose

— Helps release destructive tendencies

— Helps process and release emotional pain and self-destructive behaviors

— Provides perspective to see both sides of an issue

— Can be used for past-life healing to process abandonment and betrayal

— Encourage mutual understanding, forgiveness, and reconciliation

— Allows one to recognize their value and see their unique gifts and talents

— Enhances cooperation and community

— Instills a sense of generosity

— Encourages love for others

— Encourages forgiveness and understanding

— Releases anxiety and stress

— Protects against envy and jealousy

Nephrite Jade

Nephrite jade is revered in the East for the wisdom it provides during tranquil states. It balances masculine and feminine energies and helps heal dysfunctional relationships, while providing protection and attracting abundance. It's known as the stone of fidelity.

BENEFITS:

Increases love and nurturing

— Calms the nervous system and channels passion in healthy ways

— Supports sexual energy, fertility, and childbirth

— Heals guilt and provides confidence to overcome defeatism

— Helps one live authentically and stand out instead of adapting to fit in

— Increases trustworthiness and commitment

— Inspires love and hope later in life

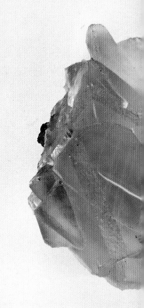

FLUORITE

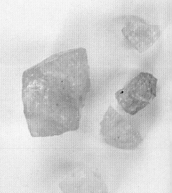

PINK BERYL

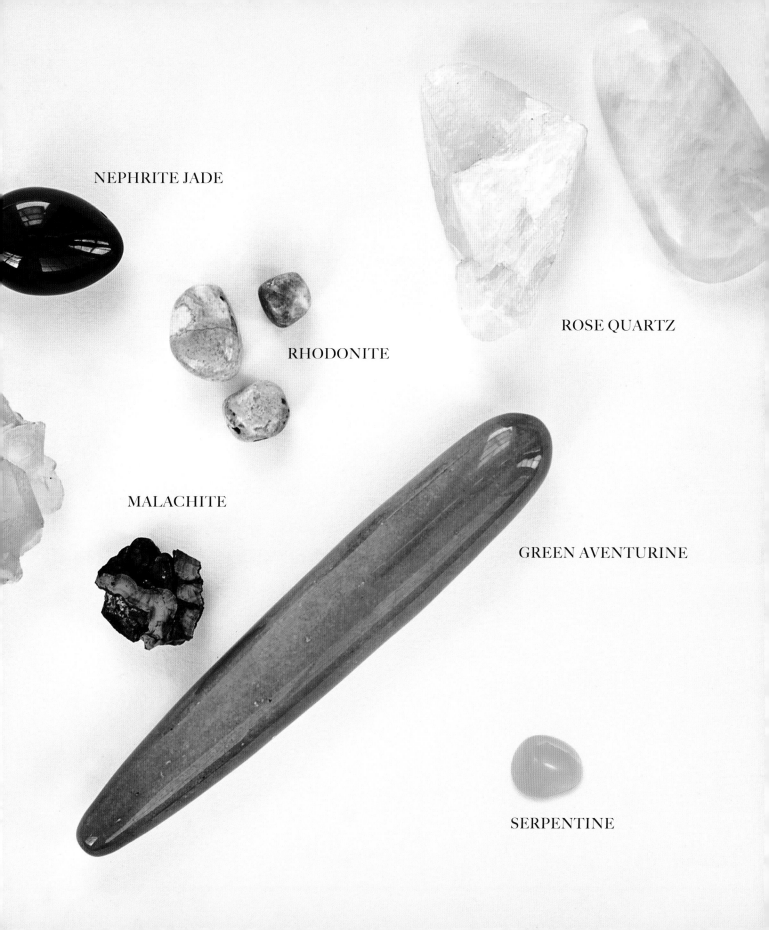

NEPHRITE JADE

RHODONITE

ROSE QUARTZ

MALACHITE

GREEN AVENTURINE

SERPENTINE

Rose Quartz

Used as a token of love as early as 600 BCE, rose quartz remains a talisman for relationships. It radiates unconditional love and strengthens bonds between friends and families. The Egyptians and Romans believed it cleared the complexion and prevented wrinkles, and rose quartz facial masks have been found in Egyptian tombs. Greek mythology claims that rose quartz was created when Aphrodite's lover Adonis was attacked by the god of war, Ares. When Aphrodite went to save him, she was caught on a briar bush, and their mingled blood stained the white quartz pink. It can be used as a powerful aphrodisiac and help one get in touch with their sensuality.

BENEFITS:

Supports connection within groups and community

— Bears a strong spiritual attunement to the Earth, Universe, and Divine

— Inspires one to nurture the self when dealing with the loss of a mother

— Stimulates sensual imagination

— Comforts and heals heart wounds

— Dissolves worries, fears, and resentments to increase the heart's ability to give and receive love

— Provides a deep sense of personal fulfillment to invite inner peace and contentment

— Helps reprogram the heart to accept love from within

— Heals emotional wounds

— Increases feelings of comfort and nurture

— Helps attract new love, romance, and intimacy

— Inspires a love of beauty and appreciation for nature

— Assists in restful sleep for adults and children and prevents nightmares or night terrors

— Can aid in reducing workplace gossip and intrusion

Malachite

Derived from the Greek word *malakos*, meaning "soft," malachite has been revered since ancient times. It was a power stone for the Egyptians, who used it to channel higher energy and increase insight by grounding it into powder and wearing it as makeup, and lining their headdresses with the stone. Malachite is an ideal stone for metaphysical purposes and will protect those who use it from negative entities. It's been called the midwife's stone, because it resonates with the female reproductive organs and treats sexual trauma. It's a flexible stone that can serve each individual differently.

BENEFITS:

Warns of danger by breaking into pieces

— Regulates the menstrual cycle and eases associated symptoms, such as cramps

— Reduces labor pain

— Helps clear and activate chakras

— Encourages loyalty and practicality in relationships

— Reveals blockages to encourage spiritual growth

— Helps process complicated emotions and makes it easier for you to break bad habits

— Encourage expression and eases social anxiety

— Provides support when dealing with anxiety and depression

— Provides courage to stand up to emotional blackmail and emotional abuse

— Promotes healthy relationships

Green Aventurine

Once used by ancient Tibetans to decorate their temples, green aventurine has been known to increase visionary powers. It provides protection to the heart chakra from negative entities who seek to prey on its energy. Known as the "stone of opportunity," green aventurine increases luck and is often used for manifestation and abundance.

BENEFITS:

Soothes emotional wounds and provides clarity to recognize issues behind imbalance, illness, depression, and other negative patterns

— Inspires lightness and humor to provide a renewed sense of optimism, joy, and hope

— Can be used as an emotional anchor to stabilize and ground

— Encourages conception when trying to get pregnant

— Amplifies leadership qualities

— Brings optimism and confidence

— Enhances appreciation for nature

— Guards against environmental pollution

— Soothes tension and strife in relationships

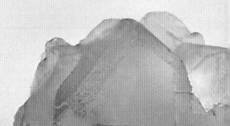

Fluorite

Fluorite has a stabilizing effect on the emotional body and provides perspective when overwhelmed or confused. It's a stone of purpose that promotes spiritual wholeness and helps one learn to quiet the chatter of the mind. Fluorite gives form and structure to energies, ideas, and concepts; stirs creativity; and opens the mind to new possibilities. As a "dream crystal," it protects the mind and is marvelous for freeing the spirit at night to explore, travel, and expand without fear or disturbance.

BENEFITS:

Helps achieve deep meditation

— Dissolves fear related to the future and making a wrong decision

— Encourages suppressed feelings to come to the surface to be resolved

— Dispels illusion and encourages flexible thinking to recognize the truth and see the big picture

— Encourages self-confidence to realize full potential

— Instills fair reasoning to help see situations objectively

— Allows relationships to flourish in a way that is beneficial for all

— Heightens intuitive powers and awakens one to how their purpose fits into the Universe's master plan

Serpentine

Derived from the Greek word *serpens* meaning snake, serpentine is a fitting name for this crystal, known for its ability to activate Kundalini energy. Ranging in color from lime to dark green, this stone is one of the few that can protect against negative energy while attracting positivity.

BENEFITS:

Attracts potential romantic partners with compatible values and interests

— Helps one achieve inner peace and assists in meditation

— Aids in breaking habits and rewiring creativity

— Encourages love and compassion in order to release aggression

— Facilitates making contact with angelic guidance

— Ancient lore claims this stone once helped nursing women regulate their milk supply

— Balances mood and encourages peaceful resolutions to conflict

Pink Beryl

Pink beryl is a crystal of the heart that can be used to attract a soulmate or deepen a current relationship. It teaches the soul how to release toxic feelings and experiences that block the heart and prevent the higher heart from opening.

BENEFITS:

Attracts abundance of love into one's life and helps maintain love as it grows

— Encourages consideration, responsibility, receptivity, and loving thoughts and actions

— Inspires joy and reverence for life

— Increases ability to experience the unconditional love of the Divine

— Helps align one's personality with the soul

— Helps one recognize unfulfilled emotional needs and feelings that need to be expressed

— Reveals fear-based defense mechanisms that block healing and transformation

— Supports girls entering puberty without their mothers

— Supports those struggling with eating disorders

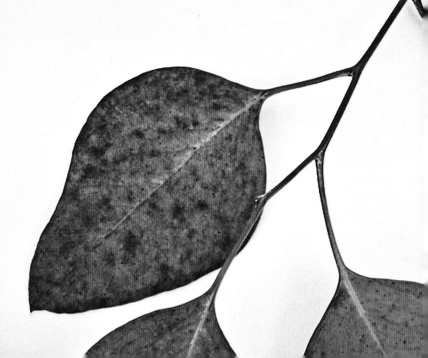

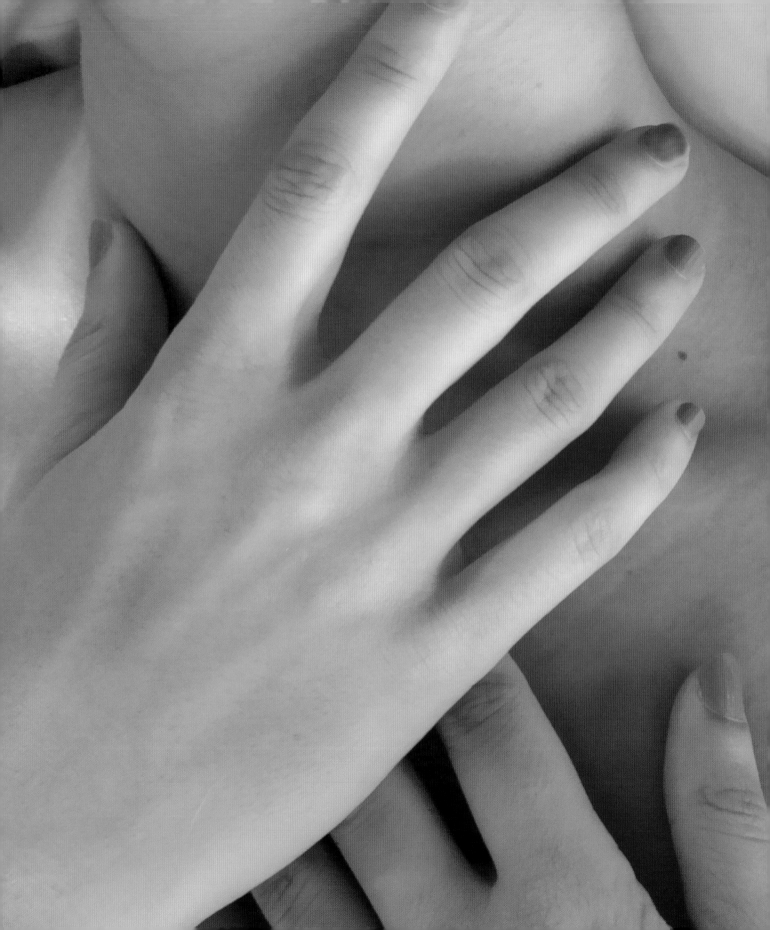

10 | THE THROAT CHAKRA

The throat chakra is located at the base of the throat, and it unlocks our ability to clearly communicate and express ourselves with ease. Here it is said that *Amrita*, a Sanskrit term defined as "the nectar of the gods" and a synonym for female ejaculation, drips down from the bindu chakra located in the front of the head. This symbolizes receiving wisdom and speaking with discernment from a place of higher knowledge.

The throat chakra is associated with the thyroid, which produces hormones that regulate metabolism, and it governs the neck, vocal chords, ears, jaws, and teeth.

A Healthy Throat Chakra

When the throat chakra is balanced, you experience ease of communication from your truest self. You have a commitment to truth, as you may experience lies as too difficult to take part in. You hold on to your intention with great focus through any obstacles. Simple pleasures are enjoyed, and comfort is found through the voices of loved ones.

When the Throat Chakra Needs Acknowledgment

If this chakra is deficient, you may find it difficult to communicate or express sexual desires and needs. Your trauma could stem from being discouraged from expressing yourself as a child. For example, being ridiculed for an appreciation of the arts, being discouraged from dressing outside of gender stereotypes, or stifling emotion can cause this chakra to be depleted.

When this chakra is in excess, you may give into idle gossip, talk too much with little self-awareness or regard for those who are forced to listen, and/or be led to compulsive behaviors such as overeating.

When this chakra is out of balance, you may experience great self-doubt. Therefore, you may not truly understand what goals to focus on, and you may even pursue other people's dreams. Without the ability to safely express yourself, you can turn to deceit to get what you want.

The Throat Chakra's Role in Communication and Creativity

When this chakra is empowered, we can communicate not just through the spoken word but non-verbally as well. We become aware of the powerful communicative powers we possess through body language, through our subtle facial expressions and overall presence.

This chakra helps us to speak our truth, not only in terms of facts but including our clarity of consciousness, our hearts, and our power. It is with this that we feel heard and that what we say resonates easier with others because it is aligned with purity.

The throat chakra is connected to the sacral chakra. The sacral is the incubator of creativity; the throat is the means to demonstrate that creativity. When it's healthy, we find it pleasurable to express our ideas and explore various aspects of our sexuality. We are active creators finding joy in expressing ourselves.

This center aligns with clarity of consciousness. When this chakra is open, we may find that we learn via speaking aloud, not afraid to hear how our words sound, and feel what resonates with our awareness. Speaking from a place of truth and listening to what is said, a person who has a healthy throat chakra will be able to feel what is right and learn from this act without judgment.

After one of her students performed well, opera teacher Renée Flemings would tell them not to try and repeat what they did or how they sang, but instead to repeat the process of how they got there. This is exactly what happens when energy flows freely in the throat chakra. Sex never becomes stagnant or about what "moves" you make. It becomes an improvised piece of art—a true creative act.

Throat Chakra Snapshot

<u>Color</u>: Pale sky blue to deep royal blue

<u>Sensual Sound</u>: *I (eye)*

<u>Musical Tone</u>: G

<u>Location</u>: Throat

<u>Governs</u>: Communication, expression

<u>Healthy</u>: Articulate, expressive, present

<u>Unhealthy</u>: Arrogant, afraid of sex, timid

<u>Sense</u>: Hearing

<u>Organ</u>: Ears

<u>Sexuality</u>: Communication, expression

<u>Element</u>: Sound

<u>Intention</u>: I Speak and Am Heard

The Sanskrit word for this chakra is *vishuddha*, meaning "purification."

Because this chakra is also tied into the sense of hearing, listening is a major component of tuning in to this energy center. Listening and allowing others to express themselves without judgment or defensiveness is another way this chakra is expressed.

Finding Your Voice:
THROAT CHAKRA PRACTICE

According to Taoist teachings, faking orgasm and pleasure, seeing sex as a performance, and anxiety can all contribute to vaginal numbness. Memories stuck in the vagina can block you from experiencing its full pleasurable potential. Take your time with this ritual. Remember, these exercises are not just about "getting off"; they are about turning on and tuning in. Whatever you experience is meant for you to experience. Keep a journal nearby to jot down any emotions, thoughts, or visions you have while performing this ritual. This will create more clarity and assurance of what you are achieving through this process of self-discovery.

For this ritual, we are going to activate and cleanse the throat chakra by internal massage, while communicating with ourselves through erotic language. This connects the sacral and throat chakras. If you do not have a vagina, you can employ the non-sensual touch elements of this exercise.

Begin by creating space for this ritual. Set it up in a place you are comfortable and will be undisturbed. Arrange it with pleasing music, scents, pillows, and/or anything else that makes you feel at ease. Thoroughly cleanse your hands and materials for this exercise.

About the G-Spot

What we call the G-spot is not a specific spot but an erogenous zone located on the upper vaginal wall halfway between the vaginal opening and the cervix. The G-spot stands out because it is surrounded by a spongy texture that swells when aroused, while the rest of the vaginal wall is smooth. The inner workings of female pleasure have only been studied in recent years, and much of the research on G-spots is conflicted, even as to its existence. Nevertheless, this mysterious hotspot has developed a reputation for producing powerful orgasms that can lead to female ejaculation.

The G-spot is surrounded by the urethral sponge, which protects the urethra and provides a safeguard to the entrance of the vagina. As arousal builds, the urethral sponge tissue fills with blood and, for some women, fluid comes out of the Skene's glands located alongside the urethra. The G-spot is not located on the front vaginal wall, but can be felt through the center or slightly to the left or right of the center of the front wall.

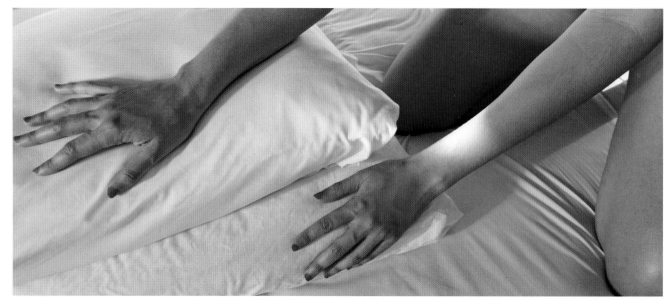

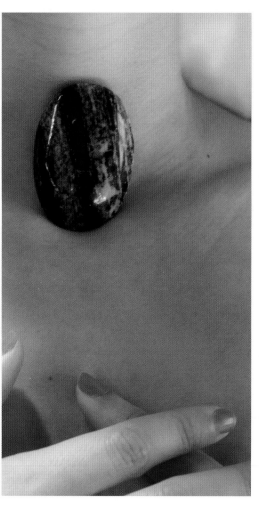

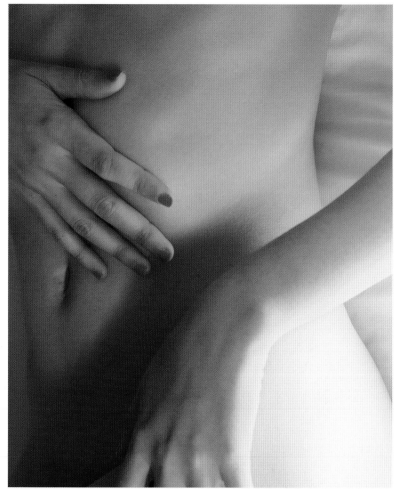

Some people are less sensitive than others are to the G-spot, and some simply won't find it arousing. Pleasure means something different to everyone, so keep an open mind about how it feels to you. But finding out means that you're pushing the boundaries of what you believed you were capable of when it comes to pleasure. Even if it doesn't end up on your "go-to" list in terms of self-pleasure, the exploration itself will lead to tapping into deeper parts of yourself.

Amrita, "the nectar of the gods," is one name for the fluid that comes out by means of female ejaculation. When you're in a state of full surrender and receptive to pleasure, this "nectar" can be fully expressed and released. It can be a lot or a little; the important thing is simply to tap into your body's amazing potential.

Choose Your Crystals

Materials

· 1 or 2 pillows

· Crystal (see pages 156 through 159)

Extras for the Throat Chakra

The throat chakra is associated with hearing. Music or soothing tones in the key of G will benefit this area. Truly tuning in and actively listening will create powerful shifts in this chakra's health.

A Rose Wand or Xaga Curve Chakrub will be curved with a bulbous tip for easily reaching the G-spot. If you don't have one, simply use your fingers and connect to a throat crystal (see page 156) by holding it in your less dominant hand over your throat chakra.

1. Undress and, laying down, place one or two pillows underneath your pelvis.

2. Place your throat chakra crystal or Chakrub on your throat chakra. Breathe deeply and tune in to the energy of the crystal. Visualize blue light shining from this area.

3. Because the throat chakra is associated with hearing and expression, you are going to speak to yourself, saying things that ignite arousal, that you would wish to hear from a lover, or what you desire to say to a significant other. Express what it is you want. Tell yourself how sexy you are, and while you say it, *hear* the words.

4. Insert your Chakrub or fingers and explore. Touch different parts of yourself and note how each feels. Use circular motions, different amounts of pressure, treating this as a massage.

5. If you are using your fingers for this exercise, you may notice that some spots feel hotter than others; this is a sign of unprocessed emotions. Send love to these areas.

6. Continue speaking through this process, expressing what it is you feel and what you want to feel. You can move onto the sensual sound for this chakra, *"eye."*

7. Whatever sensations arise internally, visualize that energy as blue filling up the throat chakra.

8. At the end of this exercise, rest with the Chakrub or throat chakra crystal on your throat chakra, and state the intention; "I feel expressive. I am heard."

If you wish to explore your G-spot, once you build up arousal, place your fingers or insert your Chakrub without using pressure. With your palm facing up, press into the front vaginal wall and make a "Come hither" motion with your fingers or Chakrub. The G-spot, when aroused, feels like the texture of a walnut shell. At first it may feel strange, but don't be afraid to press firmly.

Crystals for the Throat Chakra

The throat chakra reflects the color blue, which symbolizes trust, faith, respect, patience, and long-lasting focus to become our authentic selves and take responsibility for our actions. Light-blue crystals encourage acceptance, patience, and reconciliation when we're seeking forgiveness. They can be used to break addictions or destructive patterns, temper anger, and restore a cheerful attitude. They are ideal for coping with grief and letting go of the past. Dark-blue crystals enhance our ability to direct respect and compassion within. They pass on lessons of humanity, discretion, and being of service to others.

Blue Kyanite

Derived from the Greek word meaning "blue," kyanite is one of only a few stones that does not need to be cleansed and does not accumulate or retain negative energy. It helps one speak their truth and overcome victim mentalities. It is a highly adaptable stone and can be used for cleansing or clearing other crystals.

BENEFITS:

Encourages better communication and self-expression

— Creates a pathway for spiritual energy to flow through to thought

— Provides a path for transmitting and receiving healing energies

— Provides protection for those doing healing work

— Powerful stone for metaphysical work

— Helps one examine all aspects of the self to understand their soul's purpose

— Promotes calm and tranquility

— Reveals destructive patterns and encourages a healthy shift in perspective

— Encourages resourcefulness and logical thinking in extreme situations

— Inspires loyalty and fair treatment

— Dispels illusion, anger, and frustration

Amazonite

Amazonite is rumored to have once adorned the shields of Amazonians, a mighty tribe of female soldiers. Legend claims that some of these warriors elected to remove one breast to improve their archery skills. They would rub their wounds with a polished amazonite stone to avoid infection. It was celebrated as a stone of courage and used to heal injuries and illnesses of all kinds.

BENEFITS:

Balances masculine and feminine energies as well as parts of the personality

— Awakens compassion and allows perspective to see both sides of an issue

— Encourages acceptance of different points of view

— Aids in overcoming loneliness

— Increases self-esteem and curbs tendencies to self-neglect

— Encourages happy marriages

— Enhances effective communication and helps one choose their words wisely

— Assists in setting appropriate boundaries to establish healthy relationships

— Powerful talisman of healing and prosperity

— Treats sexual disorders such as lack of desire, impotence, and sexual obsession

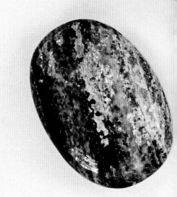

LAPIS LAZULI

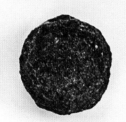

AZURITE

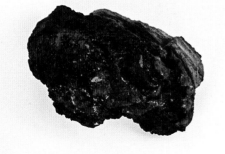

BLUE KYANITE

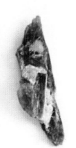

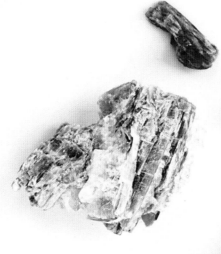

LABRADORITE

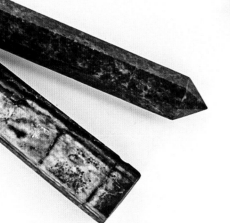

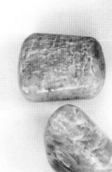

SODALITE

AMAZONITE

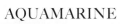

AQUAMARINE

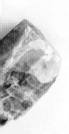

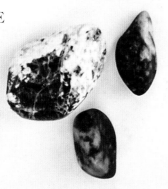

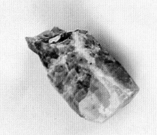

Lapis Lazuli

To the Ancient Egyptians, lapis lazuli represented the night sky and power of the gods. Adding it to medicines was thought to enhance the likelihood of being cured, what we would now consider a placebo effect. It is a crystal of universal truth and enhances all forms of communication.

BENEFITS:

Encourages honesty in both spoken and written word

— Invites calm, loving communication in homes with temperamental teenagers

— Promotes self-awareness and inner acceptance

— Allows difficult emotions to surface and releases repressed anger

— Encourages dignity in friendship and social interactions

— Provides clarity about life direction

— Reveals limitations and opportunities for growth to help one use their unique gifts

— Promotes creative problem solving

— Enhances intellectual ability and memory

— Brings harmony in relationships

— Beneficial for women suffering from menstrual irregularities

— Stimulates desire for knowledge and understanding and assists in the process of learning

Sodalite

Sodalite is called a Poet's Stone for of its ability to help one communicate profound philosophical ideas and connect the logical with the spiritual. It's a strong metaphysical stone that will help its wearer live up to their own ideas of truth and develop their intuition.

BENEFITS:

Helpful for ending arguments and communicating emotions in an honest, loving manner

— Quiets inner critic to the benefit of writers

— Encourages truthfulness within the subconscious to facilitate understanding of one's spirituality

— Encourages idealism to remain true to one's self and stand up for their beliefs

— Awakens latent creative abilities

— Stimulates psychic and clairvoyant abilities

— Illuminates negative patterns

— Strengthens the immune system

— Can be used during meditation to understand one's present situation

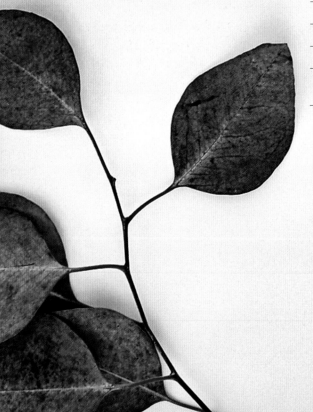

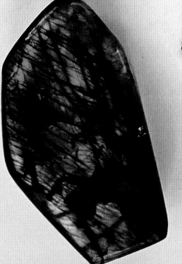

Azurite

Azurite was once considered a powerful psychic stone by the early Egyptians and settlers of Atlantis. The ancient Chinese called it the "Stone of Heaven" and believed it could open celestial gateways. It was coveted by the Greeks and Romans for its healing abilities and visionary potential. These beliefs have been passed down, and azurite is still considered a truth-enhancing, sacred stone.

BENEFITS:

Helps break negative patterns that stem from insecurity and fear

— Can be used to explore past or alternate lives and the ability to communicate the lessons from such experiences

— Invites healing light into consciousness and infuses it in thoughts, feelings, words, and actions

— Helps release stress and worry and provides courage to overcome grief and sadness

— Reveals reasons behind fears and phobias to facilitate their release

— Ideal for overcoming inferiority complexes and overcoming domestic bullying

— Provides confidence to those who hold back from expressing themselves

— Able to move subconscious thought to the front of the mind, where it can be tested for truth

— Protects one from being misled and allows them to decipher the truth

— Calms those who speak out of nervousness

Labradorite

The ancient Inuit believed that labradorite fell from the frozen fire of the Aurora Borealis, explaining its extraordinary shimmer, which seems to separate our waking world from that of the unseen. Considered the matriarch of the subconscious mind, labradorite continues to be revered by spiritual shamans, healers, and divinators for its abilities to enhance intuition and connect us with higher realms.

BENEFITS:

Enables one to understand an energy field without entering it or absorbing its conditions

— Reduces anti-social, reckless, and impulsive behavior

— Provides moral strength for those who are easily led by others

— Awakens a sense of adventure to remove the emotional drain of daily routine and responsibility

— Protects from negativity and misfortune

— Assists in communication with higher realms

— Uplifts while banishing fears and enhancing trust in the universe

— Merges intellectual thought with intuitive wisdom to dispel illusion and understand the root causes of issues

— Energizes the imagination

— Enhances faith and reliance on one's self

— Beneficial for uniting the chakra system

Aquamarine

The oceanic blue reflected in aquamarine evokes calmness and relaxation, and it was once believed to be the treasure of mermaids. Sailors carried it as a talisman of safe travel and good luck. It was believed to be a stone of eternal youth.

BENEFITS:

Moves heart energy upward to allow one to speak their deepest, heartfelt truths

— Empowering stone that reveals the power in yielding instead of using force

— Provides courage to women to listen to their inner voice and enhance their intuition

— Dispels emotional numbness to allow men to communicate their feelings more easily

— Cleanses the emotional body and opens communication

— Gently brings emotional patterns to the surface to understand limitations

— Helps identify where the ego is causing one to play the victim or overreacting

— Provides support to children who have been through traumatic experiences and have disassociated from their emotional bodies

— Helps in moving through transition and change and reduces resistance to the unknown

— Helps clear out emotional baggage

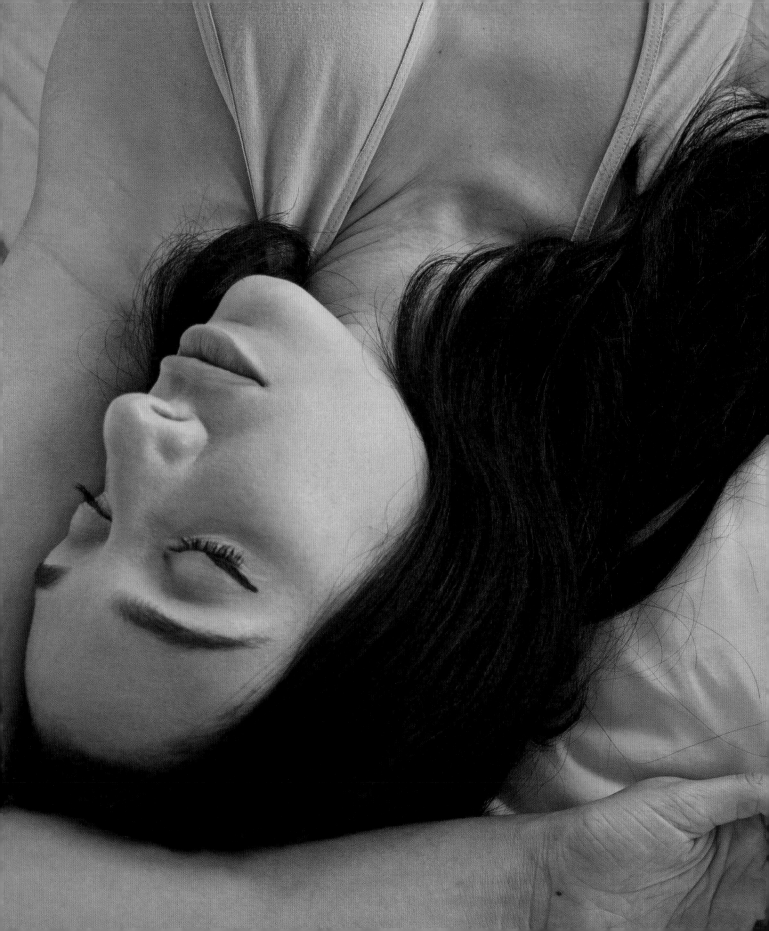

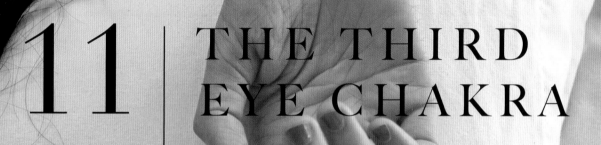

11 | THE THIRD EYE CHAKRA

The third eye chakra, sometimes referred to as the "brow chakra," is located at the top of the spinal column, inside the pineal gland. It is with this chakra that we learn to ascend from individuality, transcend duality, and enhance our inner and psychic sight.

Physically, this chakra governs the autonomic nervous system, which regulates primarily unconscious bodily functions such as heart rate. The pituitary gland, which produces critical hormones such as cortisol, is also associated with the third eye chakra. This chakra manages the neurological system, the brain, and the eyes.

The pea-sized pituitary gland, located behind the forehead between the eyes, is often called the "seat of the mind" because it controls emotional as well as concrete thoughts. It is responsible for various bodily functions and produces critical hormones, including oxytocin. Also known as the "love hormone," oxytocin is a natural antidepressant that promotes intimate bonding and is released when we orgasm, during childbirth, and while breastfeeding. Two people who share a strong sexual attraction will produce more oxytocin hormone than two who do not, which explains why feelings sometimes develop quickly after we have sizzling sex with someone new.

A Healthy Third Eye Chakra

When your third eye chakra is in balance, you have a sense of ease when faced with problems, and you find joy in solving them. Your intellect and intuition are married. When this chakra is balanced, your imagination is used positively. You have a strong understanding of what motivates you and other people, and you can determine what needs to be done when something isn't flowing correctly in life.

You are connected to the flow and synchronicities of life. You may be proficient in interpreting "signs," and you may even have psychic perceptions. You can find guidance in your dreams.

When the Third Eye Chakra Needs Acknowledgment

When this chakra is deficient, you may express co-dependency due to a lack of trust in your own ability to understand. You may often have mental fog and confusion. You may be in denial about relationship issues or be deceived easily, not wanting to "see" the truth. When this chakra is in excess, you may give into fantasizing often, without the grounding element of putting dreams into reality. You may give into overthinking, become easily frustrated, and struggle to think outside of the box.

Other Body Experiences with the Third Eye Chakra

Tapping into this chakra sexually can be quite interesting. The third eye gives us the ability to perceive things outside of our physical reality. The sexuality of this chakra is vision, and when it's imbalanced, a person may have strong affinities toward pornography or be very appearance-minded when finding a mate.

When nurtured, the extra-sensory perception of vision can enable you to experience your partner's feelings, removing barriers of perceived genders. If you choose, you may dissolve the physical understanding of your sexual pleasure and move onto sensing what it feels like with other genitalia. This is due to the chakra's ability to see through insight and the ability to visualize structures through essence of anything's inherent makeup. The awareness that we are all a manifestation of one spirit occurs in this chakra.

The archetype associated with this chakra is the Intuitive—one who can call upon information from extrasensory places. Think of the Intuitive as opposed to the Intellectual, who comes across as cold and arrogant.

Third Eye Chakra Snapshot

Color: Indigo, deep purple

Sensual Sound: *Ay*

Musical Tone: A

Location: Third eye

Governs: Intuition

Healthy: Wise, master of self, charismatic

Unhealthy: Manipulative

Sense: No predominant sense

Organ: Mind

Sexuality: Visual/vision

Element: Light

Intention: I See

Lucid Dreams

Lucid dreams are dreams in which you are aware that you are dreaming. The official definition in The American Psychological Association's *2007 Dictionary of Psychology* is, "a dream in which the sleeper is aware that he or she is dreaming and may be able to influence the progress of the dream narrative."

Becoming familiar with this type of dream allows the dreamer to gain more conscious control in the dreamscape. Doing so can have benefits; you may be able to ask your subconscious for advice, for example, or live out a fantasy that you may not be able to in waking life. Feeling liberated from waking-state limitations can bring joy and a sense of freedom. Lucid dreams can also help expose areas of life that may be stagnant due to self-limiting beliefs and emotions that need to be processed.

The book *Erotic Spirituality* explains, "Similarly, one will be told that erotic sculpture has nothing to do with sex, except insofar as sex itself, like battle, may be employed as a symbolism of higher things." Understanding what desires come about in our lucid dreams can show what we symbolically desire to feel in waking life, or it can simply pinpoint untapped sexual desires that we have not been able to express.

Eleventh-century Buddhist sage Naropa named dream yoga one of the Six Yogas of Naropa, his accelerated path to enlightenment. With this unique state of sentience, one may experience the essence of non-duality—the implication of a healthy functioning third eye chakra. Lucid dreaming can be a great tool for connecting your consciousness and your subconscious for greater alignment. Whether you want to live out sexual fantasies, create emotional healing, or enhance your inner guidance system, lucid dreaming can be a powerful tool in your toolbox.

Everyone dreams each night, but dream recall varies depending on many factors. To increase your chances of having a lucid dream, first increase your dream recall. When you wake up in the morning, immediately ask yourself if you remember what you've dreamt. You may even wish to keep a piece of paper by your bedside that says, "Did I dream?" or set your alarm to ask this question. Write down anything you remember. Over time, your dream recall will become stronger.

One way to increase probability of a lucid dream is to put marks on your hands with a marker. Throughout the day, when you see these marks, ask yourself, "Am I dreaming?" You will eventually ask yourself the same thing in your sleeping state. When the answer is yes, you will empower yourself to go forth with your lucid dream work. You could also try drinking Valerian root tea, which is known to induce lucid dreaming. For this section, we include a list of crystals that are known to benefit dream recall and lucid dreaming.

Word Origin: Third Eye Chakra

The Sanskrit word for this chakra is *Ajna*, which means "summoning" or "unlimited power." It is so named because this is the energy center from which all chakras are guided.

Summoning the Power of Dreams:
THIRD EYE CHAKRA EXERCISE

When we connect to the third eye chakra, we can experience sexuality in our mind's eye, using our imagination to fulfill unmet fantasies, and we can receive insight into hidden desires we may not be aware of consciously. To do this, we will work on promoting intentional lucid dreaming through the aid of a crystal.

This practice is repeated over time. It starts with dream recall as often as possible. Meditating or sleeping with the crystals under your pillow can offer support to this process.

Disclaimer: Lucid dreaming is a powerful tool for gaining insight and creative problem solving, but those suffering from depression, feelings of disassociation, or mental illness should consult a therapist or physician before engaging in this practice.

Materials

· Bed
· Crystal (see page 166)
· Notebook

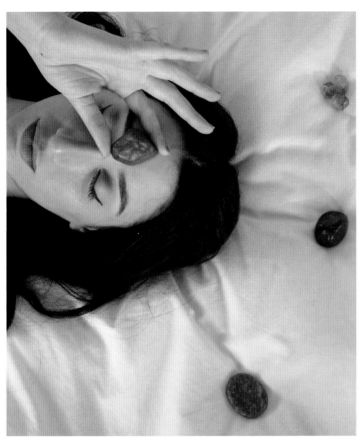

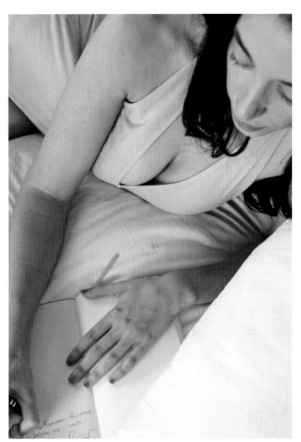

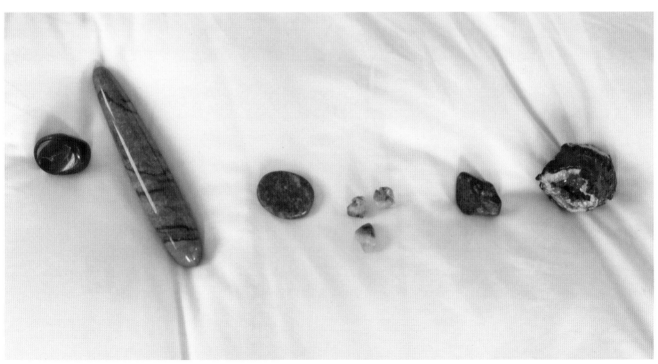

Choose Your Crystals

Keeping one of these crystals under your pillow may enhance dreams. For this exercise, you can also include a third eye crystal for stronger effects.

Stichtite: Found in shades of hot pink to deep purple, stichtite can be used as a link between the heart and higher brow and crown chakras. It is a powerful stone that can be used for enhancing spiritual connection and dream interpretation. Incorporate it in a dreamcatcher or place it under your pillow to help capture your dream essence.

Phenacite: Phenacite is a high-vibration stone that exudes pure white light. It is considered by many to be the highest-energy crystal on the planet. It can be used to stimulate visionary intuition and telepathic abilities and to heal the chakras.

Scolecite: Scolecite is a high-vibration stone that can open up communication with your higher self. It aids in achieving inner peace and spiritual transformation and is excellent for meditation. Scolecite may help you relax deeply into restful sleep and tune in to the messages from your dreams.

Ametrine: A mixture of the quartz crystals amethyst and citrine, ametrine enhances spiritual clarity and creativity. It activates the third eye chakra and can be used for astral travel, dreams, and meditation. It helps connect the spiritual realm with day-to-day life.

Moldavite: Formed 20 million years ago when meteors crashed into Earth, moldavite is a stone of connectivity and carries an intense frequency. The impact of the meteorites caused the existing rock material to melt and fuse with the meteor material, creating a new crystal with earthly and extraterrestrial energies. It stimulates the heart, brow, and crown chakras and is a powerful aide for meditation and dream work. Moldavite can be used to improve telepathic sensitivities, channeling, and cosmic consciousness.

Lepidolite: Lepidolite is a calming crystal that promotes balance, relaxation, and peaceful sleep. Because it contains lithium, lepidolite can also be used to treat mild anxiety and for stress relief. It helps activate your connection to your higher self and can be used for dreamwork and recall. Lepidolite works well with all the chakras, but it is especially well-suited to the higher chakras.

Extras for the Third Eye Chakra

Your imagination is a powerful tool for increasing the strength of your third eye. Take some time to perform some mental exercises that work outside of typical constructs: Imagine you are seeing the world from a bird's view. Imagine you are expanding and growing. Imagine you are smaller than an ant. Visualization opens up the mind to creative experiences that can expand your conscious awareness.

Azurite: The rich blue of azurite resonates at the exact frequency of the third eye chakra. Ancient Egyptian, Native American, Chinese, Greek, and Roman cultures all revered azurite for its powerful metaphysical properties. It is good for meditation, aids psychic awareness, and increases intuition. It can be used to enhance dreams or enter trance states, and it is beneficial for exploring past lives.

Quartz: Quartz is the most common crystal on the planet and can be found in a range of colors. Despite its wide availability, clear quartz is far from average. It is known as the "stone of power" and amplifies any energy or intention. It is extremely beneficial for manifesting, healing, meditation, protection, and channeling. Smoky quartz is ideal for treating insomnia, nightmares, and hyperactivity. Agate can also be used for bad dreams. A newly discovered type of quartz called Dream Quartz, which originates in Colombia, contains prehnite and epidote and can assist in lucid dreaming or astral projection.

Amethyst: Amethyst is a calming stone that aids in dream recollection and promotes peaceful sleep and serenity. The ancient Greeks and Romans believed amethyst to be a stone of sobriety, and they made drinking gourds from it believing that would prevent intoxication. Amethyst allows us to release control to receive messages from the spiritual realm.

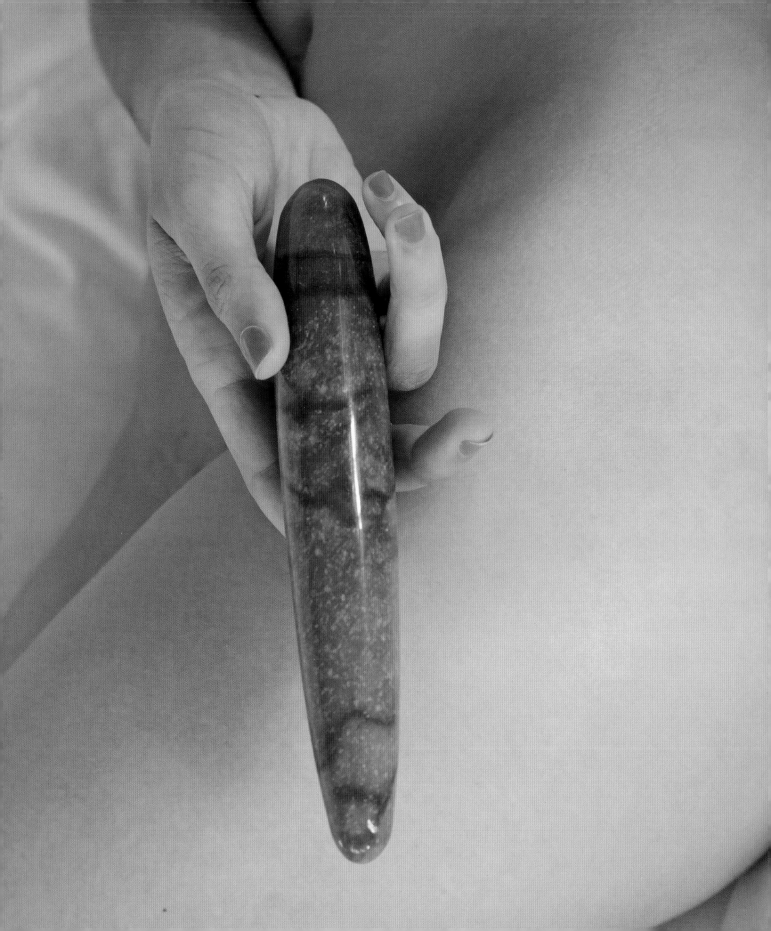

1. Before bed, sit up in a comfortable position.

2. Hold your crystal(s) in your less dominant hand.

3. Breathe and relax.

4. Visualize a golden light surrounding you, with the intention of only good energy coming in and only good energy going out.

5. Tune in to the energy of the crystal and breathe in its energy.

6. With your dominant hand, place the crystal in front of your third eye.

7. Visualize beautiful indigo light shining in this area.

8. Repeat the following suggestion: "Tonight during my sleep, I will have a lucid dream that will allow me to _____." Fill in the blank with your intention. For example, it could be "fulfill my fantasy of same-sex experience," "reveal blockages that I may not be aware of," or "restore health and well-being so I wake up feeling refreshed and energized."

9. Place the crystal under your pillow or next to your bed and repeat your intention while falling asleep.

High levels of excitement during lucid dreaming may cause the dream to end. Practicing stabilizing your emotions. When you become aware that you are dreaming, follow these guidelines:

1. Be aware of your emotions and mentally tell yourself to calm down to reduce feelings of excitement.

2. Focus your visual attention on something boring, such as your hands or any emotionally neutral scene.

3. Concentrate on one simple task at a time.

Write down your dreams when you wake up. If problems arose in them, ask yourself, "Do I feel this way in any area of my waking life?" and "What would I do to feel better about how this dream ended?" Through practicing this insight into your subconscious, you will begin to gain that insight for issues that arise in your waking life. Recognizing your subconscious as an internal guidance system will allow you to seek your inner wisdom to gain new perspectives and build trust with your intuition.

Lucid dreaming can have a profound impact on your waking life. It allows you to rehearse for real-life situations, process grief, practice a physical skill, and train emotional responses. Lucid dreaming can also be a source of inspiration and help you get in touch with your higher self.

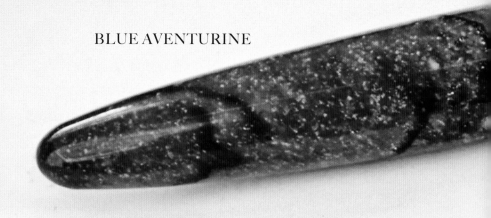

BLUE AVENTURINE

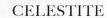

BLUE AVENTURINE

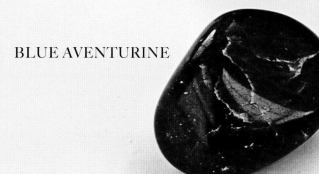

CELESTITE

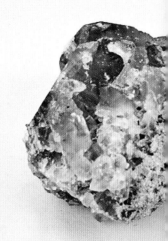

Crystals for the Third Eye

The third eye chakra is represented by a soft shade of indigo. Crystals of this color will encourage introspection and can help immensely in the quest for knowledge. Indigo stones combine the intuition of violet with the trust and honest of pure blue, helping pave the way to a higher plane of consciousness. Indigo stones encourage present-moment awareness and help bring understanding to complex relationships.

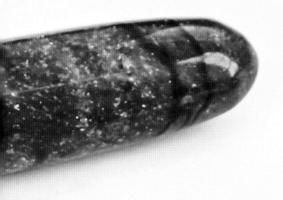

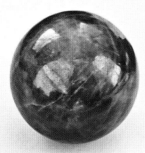

IOLITE

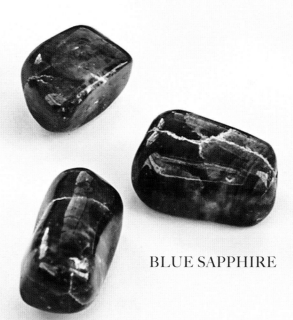

BLUE SAPPHIRE

DUMORTIERITE

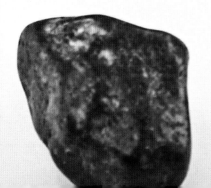

Blue Aventurine

To the ancient Tibetans, blue aventurine symbolized visionary powers and was used to improve nearsightedness as well as enhance creativity. It combines the elements of wind and water to work calmly and rationally within the heart and the mind.

BENEFITS:

Beneficial in overcoming bad habits and negative personality traits

— Encourages maturation to take responsibility for one's life and relationships
— Balances hormones and supports healthy blood
— Increases abundance, opportunities, and luck
— Enhances psychic and intuitive abilities
— Provides self-discipline and inner strength
— Helps one make clear decisions and commit to them
— Calms fiery emotions and allows one to be less affected by external influences
— Enhances masculine energy
— Calms a troubled spirit and brings about peace

Blue Sapphire

An ancient stone of royalty, blue sapphire signifies wisdom, structure, discipline, and strength. This stone has the power to transform negative thoughts and encourage acceptance and healing.

BENEFITS:

Empowers us to break free from self-imposed prisons and psychic suffering that makes us shut down emotionally

— Releases depression and lightens the mood
— Provides strength to those who are easily swayed by others' opinions
— Brings a calm focus to the mind and restores balance in the body
— Promotes understanding of the self and builds confidence to express one's truths
— Excellent for healing an inferiority complex
— Used as a symbol of love, commitment, and fidelity
— Fosters attachment and could prolong connections or cause bitter feelings
— Helps one remain committed to their spiritual path and promotes self-discipline
— Encourages the mind to open to beauty and intuition

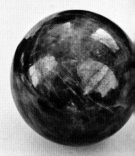

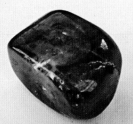

Celestite

Celestite comes from the Greek word meaning "celestial," for its pale blue color. It is a powerful stone used for cosmic connection, dream recollection, and out-of-body experiences.

BENEFITS:

May discourage certain genetic disorders from taking hold by turning on positive genetic potential and restoring order to the cell

— Provides clarity in the midst of chaotic circumstances and helps one overcome traumatic periods

— Lends support to performers as it alleviates stage fright and nervousness

— Restores balance and harmony and helps one maintain inner peace

— Heightens divine intuition and can be useful for Reiki practitioners

— Facilitates deep meditation states and opens the mind to communication from higher realms

— Enables dreamer to recall information from dreams with greater detail and clarity

— Improves dysfunctional relationships by creating space for peaceful negotiation

— Purifies the auras of all beings

— Provides emotional protection and enable release of negative energy held in the emotional body

Iolite

Iolite is a mysterious crystal that some believe was used by the Vikings as a compass to navigate sea voyages. The beautiful indigo shade of iolite resonates with the energy of twilight and stimulates astral bodies and psychic awareness. This is an ideal stone for astrologers, tarot readers, and other intuitives.

BENEFITS:

Reveals realms beyond waking consciousness and can be used for increasing visionary abilities and past- and alternate-life work

— Allows one to access thoughts and ideas beyond the ordinary to engage their creative mind

— Awakens and supports one's psychic gifts

— Examines the inner path of the deep self and allows one to release control over inner experiences

— Increases ability to move forward and heal past wounds

— Helps one recover the lost parts of the self and achieve spiritual peace

— Provides solutions to difficult problems and calms the mind to make rational decisions

— Balances the masculine and feminine aspects of one's personality

— Heals relationship issues and helps overcome co-dependency by allowing one to take responsibility for their life and happiness

— Excellent for shamanic journeying and increases the vividness and detail of inner visions

Dumortierite

Dumortierite is an ideal stone for grounding during spiritual work and enhances intellectual abilities. It amplifies one's spiritual gifts and aides those working in psychic fields of employment to relay messages with accuracy.

BENEFITS:

Helps one remember their soul

— Instills confidence in the self and abilities

— Helps one overcome mindsets related to poverty and sexual trauma that have arisen from past lives of chastity

— Allows one to see how the soul's previous purpose no longer serves and embrace the lessons of this soul's lifetime

— Allows one to acquire many psychic gifts

— Can help break patterns and overcome addictions

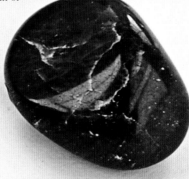

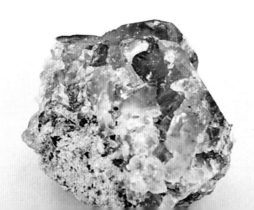

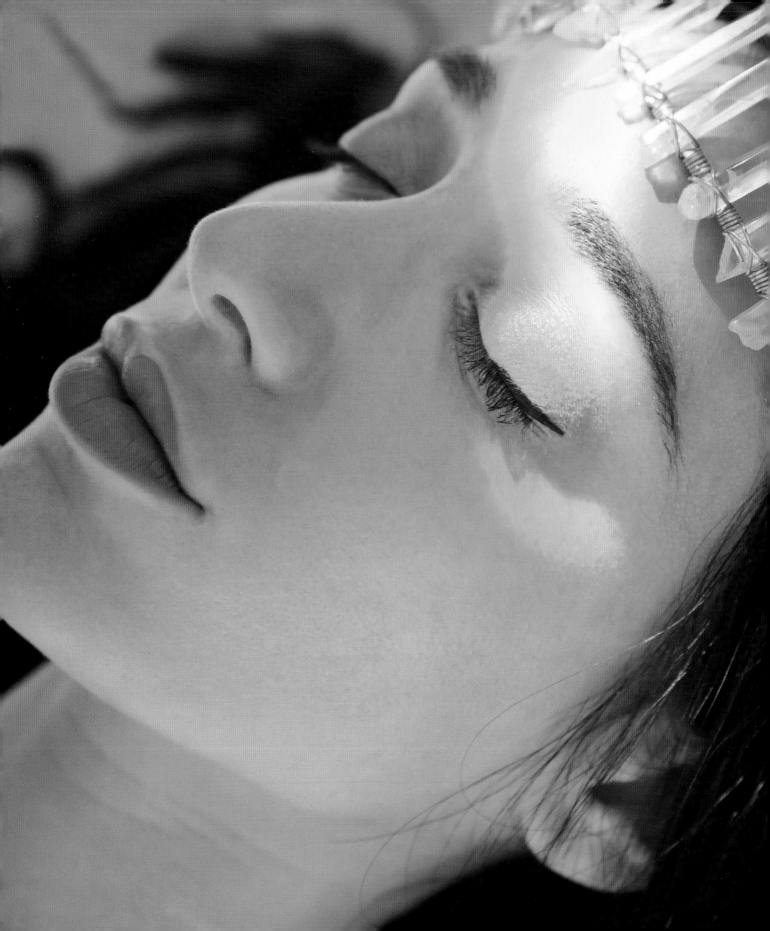

12 | THE CROWN CHAKRA

The crown chakra is on top of the head, allowing us to connect to universal consciousness. This chakra allows us to comprehend that we are all one, and it strengthens our relationship to divination.

Physically this chakra governs the skull and the brain. It is associated with the central nervous system, cerebral cortex, pineal gland, and hypothalamus. Our ability to learn new information and our mental health have a lot to do with the functionality of the crown chakra.

A Healthy Crown Chakra

A healthy and balanced crown chakra allows sexual experiences to feel profound and enables one to feel in union with source energy, otherwise known as ecstasy. Egotism is lost here, as the experience of being connected to something great encapsulates you into a feeling of purpose. You'll better understand your place both in the world and on your spiritual journey.

A feeling of bliss stems from connection to this chakra. You'll experience a quiet yet powerful understanding of the bigger picture—why everything is as it is. The ability to honor past romantic relationships for what they have taught you and compassion for those who have hurt you are also strengthened through working with this energy center.

It is when connected to this chakra that we feel open to experiencing sexuality outside of our physical bodies, opening us up to energetic orgasms—orgasms that don't require genital stimulation.

Crown Chakra Snapshot

Color: Pale lilac through lavender to deep purple

Secondary Color: White

Sensual Sound: *Ee*

Musical Tone: B

Location: Top of head

Governs: Spiritual attunement

Healthy: Spiritually connected, knowing without thought or reason

Unhealthy: Destructive sexual expression, depression

Sexuality: Spiritual experiences

Element: Thought

Intention: I Know and Understand

When the Crown Chakra Needs Acknowledgment

Word Origin: Crown Chakra

The Sanskrit name for this center is *Sahasrara*, meaning "thousand."

If this chakra has deficiencies, you may experience a lack of purpose. You may look to your romantic partner as an authority figure, and place grand illusions on yourself, celebrities, or partners. This could be because of a lack of connectedness to source energy, or "that which you call god," as you may place emphasis on materialistic items or people to fill that void. You may experience a lack of self-trust or feelings of spiritual abandonment.

If this chakra has excesses, you may seem to float on air, as you aren't grounded, and you may become addicted to fantastical spiritual ideas. The materialism of spirituality—having a certain fashion sense, decorating a particular way, or hoarding new age trends, for example—is expressed when this chakra is imbalanced. You might view past relationships through a mentality of entitlement, placing full blame on the other person, giving them authority in order to fill a spiritual void.

Loneliness is a natural part of the human experience. But connecting to the crown chakra and feeling that sense of connectedness to source energy allows us to recall that we are not alone; we are all connected. In this way, we allow the energy of loneliness to flow through us, rather than become solidified as isolation.

Royalty of the Crown Chakra

Think of a crown, with its pointy golden shape, being a conduit of powers beyond our physical senses. It has royalty and grace—royalty in the sense that we are connected to higher realms of consciousness, and grace because it is not met with egotism. This understanding puts us in alignment with values of interconnectedness. It helps us to understand that all the events of our lives are opportunities for higher learning.

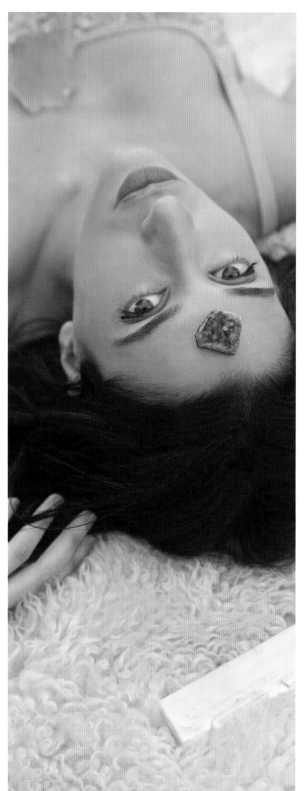

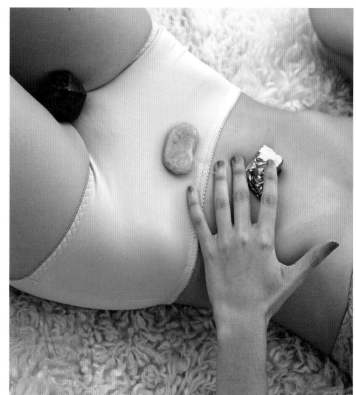

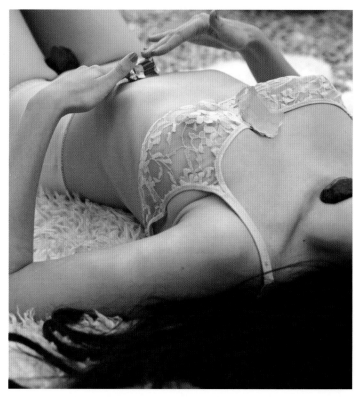

Energy Orgasm:
CROWN CHAKRA EXERCISE

For this exercise, you will be opening up to experiencing an energy orgasm. Unlike a clitoral or G-spot orgasm, energy or breath orgasms don't require physical stimulation to occur (though they can happen in conjunction). I first experienced something like this in a workshop given by Barbara Carrellas. When she demonstrated it, she had a giggle fit. That was what her energy orgasm looked like—laughing harder and harder until it reached an energetic pique and then relaxing. My energy orgasm caused me to cry (as soon as the energy reached my heart chakra). It was an instant release. It could happen for you as a very subtle feeling, or you may experience it in a much larger way. Be patient and remain open to experiencing whatever you're meant to. The more time you spend building up energy in each area, the more intense it will be.

This technique is inspired by the Fire Breath Orgasm, taught by Harley "SwiftDeer" Reagan, founder of the Deer Tribe Metis Medicine Society. According to Harley, fire breath orgasm was first done in ceremony by the Cherokee and is an important aspect of sex education and healing. Additional variations of fire breath orgasm have been found in ancient tantric and Taoist texts.

Eating clean for the day, exercising, or doing yoga will also prepare you to feel this more intensely. Fasting and detoxifying can also be beneficial for this chakra; however, consult a medical professional about the types of fasting and detoxes that will work best for you.

This exercise takes place with you lying flat on your back, so choose a space where you are comfortable lying on the floor. It is best to practice this on a hard surface (not cushiony like a bed). Lay down a blanket or yoga mat. If you have neck or back injuries, you may wish to grab added pillows to cushion them.

Pick a time when you will not be interrupted for at least an hour. You may choose to fill the area with sage, copal, myrrh, frankincense, juniper, or palo santo, or spray it with essential oils. You can put on instrumental music or music that is in a foreign language so you are not distracted by understanding the lyrics.

Set an intention for this practice. When you're working with the crown chakra, being that it is a portal to divine realms and a channel for spiritual awakening, your intention may be simply, "I know and understand." If you'd like, you can add onto this intention with something more specific to you and what you are feeling called to increase your faith in.

Choose Your Crystals

Crystals that are violet, white, clear, or golden are excellent for working with the crown chakra. A point or wand is beneficial, as in this exercise we are moving energy from the root chakra up to the crown chakra. Now that you have a crystal that corresponds to each chakra, you can place each one on its corresponding center on your body.

Optional: Keep a piece of black tourmaline by your feet to remain grounded throughout this exercise.

Lay down flat on your back with your knees bent and your feet flat on the floor. Place each of your chakra crystals on the seven chakras with the root chakra crystal on your pubic bone and your crown chakra crystal about two inches above your head. If any crystals fall during this practice, gently place them back. This exercise will take about 20 minutes.

1. Get comfortable and focus on your breathing. Take note of any tension you are holding in your body and let it go. Take your time and continue until you feel clear in your mind and relaxed in your body.

2. Breathe more deeply. Open your mouth and release all the air from your lungs. Then, slowly breathe as much air in through your nose as you can. At the height of this breath, take in a little more. Release it slowly through your mouth. At the bottom of the breath, see if you can release a little more. Do this again, and again, and again. In through the nose, out through the mouth. Take no pauses; just make it a continuous circular breathing pattern.

3. Bring attention to your root chakra and tap this crystal with your dominant hand. You may wish to add sensual touch by also moving your hands over your thighs, or do whatever feels good. Imagine the feeling of intense pleasure and visualize it being released from tapping the crystal. Infuse erotic energy into your breathing and contractions. On an exhale, you can moan the root chakra sensual sound "uh."

4. When you feel the energy in this area has built to its highest potential, begin tapping your sacral chakra crystal. Energy follows thought forms, so simply think about pulling energy from the earth into your perineum. Let energy brew in your root and sacral chakras; imagine it circulating back and forth. As this area begins to light up, move your attention to the solar plexus chakra by tapping its corresponding crystal. Allow the energy to move from your root up through your belly, then from your sacral chakra to your solar plexus. Keep circulating and letting the fire build.

Materials

· Crystal(s) (see pages 182 through 185)

· Pillows or cushions

Extras for the Crown Chakra

It is normal for energy levels to fluctuate during this practice. If your energy dips, simply return to the area where it began to dwindle and start again. Tap into your sexual center and clench your pelvic floor (PC) muscles to reactivate that energy. One of the key aspects to learning this technique is to believe that it is possible. It can sound far-fetched to someone who hasn't witnessed it firsthand, and it is often best learned by watching someone else practice it.

If your PC muscles start to cramp, try squeezing every three or four breaths instead of on every inhale.

5. Next move your attention up and tap the heart chakra crystal. Circulate energy from the belly to the heart, back and forth.

6. As you work your way up from the heart to the throat chakra, you might find yourself making some noises. If this does not happen automatically, consciously make sounds to help clear energy and allow it to move through the higher chakras. The sensual sound associated with the crown chakra is "ee". Keep circulating energy between the heart and throat chakras until you can feel it rising to the third eye.

7. Distribute energy from the throat to the third eye, continuously tapping the crystals and visualizing orgasmic energy being released.

8. Move the energy from the third eye to the crown of your head. It might feel like energy is shooting from the top of your head, like water out of a spigot. Let it flow through you. Your breathing patterns will change, your heart rate may quicken, and you might laugh hysterically or cry. With practice, you'll learn to ride these waves of energetic pleasure.

9. At the end of this practice, ground your body into the floor by pressing your weight against it. Disperse the energy you've created around your entire body, resume to a normal breathing pattern, and state your intention: "I am understanding more and more."

If any crystals fall during this practice, gently place them back. You can also keep them by your side and use the ones you need for whichever correlating chakra you are working on. You can also employ one crystal and move it as you work up towards the crown.

Whatever your experience, don't get discouraged. What comes up from you is meant for you. Whether you have an energy orgasm or not, note that you are learning to be aware of energy and beginning to incorporate that understanding into your life. Try to be patient. Some people will achieve orgasm on their first try, and for others it may take years. Continue practicing even if you do not experience an orgasm. The breathing and energy techniques involved in this practice will help to remove blocks so that orgasmic energy can flow through you. Blocks can be experienced in a variety of ways—stress, frustration, crying, or the surfacing of old memories, for example. Just breathe through it. Imagine yourself releasing old stagnant energy with each exhale and bringing in new energy with each inhale.

CHAROITE

AMETHYST

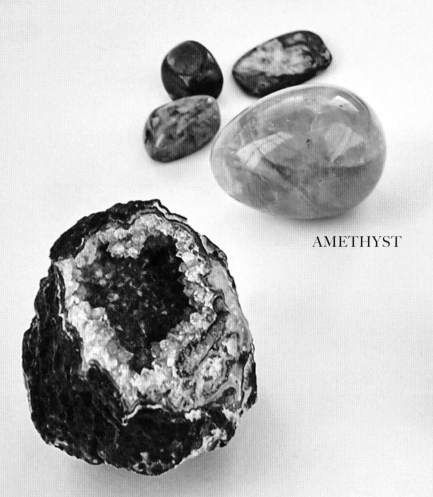

AMETHYST

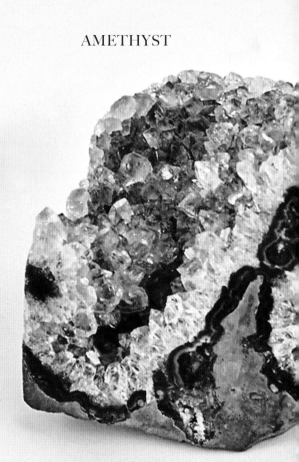

Crystals for the Crown Chakra

The crown chakra's primary color is violet, and its secondary color is white. Violet crystals awaken the intuition, enhance dreams, and stir the imagination. It is also the color of nobility and luxury and evokes pleasure. White crystals reflect the energy of the moon, natural cycles, birth, and regeneration. Just as the moon was once our guiding light during the dark hours, white crystals can illuminate the unseen spiritual world.

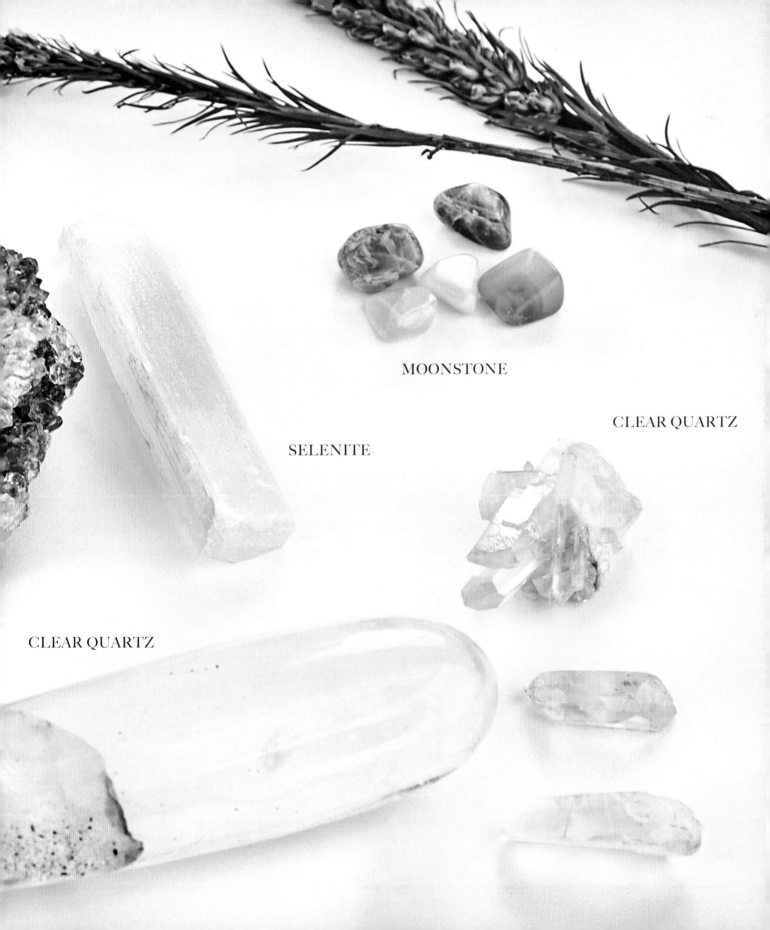

MOONSTONE

CLEAR QUARTZ

SELENITE

CLEAR QUARTZ

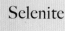

Selenite

Named after the Greek moon goddess Selene, one eleventh-century lapidary claimed that selenite grew with the waxing moon and diminished with the waning phases. It is one of few stones that does not need to be cleansed and can be used to cleanse other stones or objects. A crystallized version of gypsum, which is used for luck and protection, Selenite will dissolve in water. Desert rose selenite can be used to dissolve self-imposed limitations and assist in replacing those programs.

BENEFITS:

Encourages mental flexibility and honesty to help maintain loving relationships with ease

— Good for the spinal column, puberty, menopause, joints, and breasts

— Encourages harmony and inner peace, allowing one to recognize love and act in a loving manner

— Promotes fertility and increases the libido, provides protection during pregnancy and menopause

— Shields the mind from negative influences

— Acts as an emotional stabilizer and cures mood swings

— Brings divine light to everything it touches and transmutes emotional energy

— Releases feelings behind psychosomatic illnesses and emotional blockages

— Helps one understand inner processes and integrate shadow qualities

— Helps connect to higher self, guides, and past lives

— Strengthens memory

— Reverses the effects of free radicals

— Clears energy blockages

— Assists with meditation

— Promotes fertility and increases the libido

— Promotes mental clarity

— Enhances the properties of other stones and ideal for crystal grids

Moonstone

Ancient Romans believed the highly coveted moonstone encapsulated the image of Diana, the Moon Goddess, who could endow love, wealth, victory, and wisdom upon its possessor. Moonstone contains as many mysteries as the moon and is a crystal of love and eroticism that promotes fertility. A moonstone necklace worn during lovemaking at the full moon is believed to harmonize the body into the natural lunar cycle.

BENEFITS:

Attunes one to the natural rhythms of the body and enables natural energy cycles

— Promotes ease in pregnancy and childbirth, alleviates menstrual problems, and balances the hormonal system

— Stimulates Kundalini energy and carnal desires

— Helps reunite loved ones who have parted in anger

— Opens the heart to nurturing qualities to allow one to accept love

— Encourages mastery of emotions by bringing them under control of the higher will rather than repressing them

— Identifies emotional patterns stored in the subconscious

— Enhances the intuitive side of the mind and helps women claim their feminine power and clairvoyant abilities

— Assists men in becoming more in tune with their feminine nature and encourages creative, non-linear thinking

— Soothing for those spending the night away from home; drives away nightmares and encourages restful sleep

— Treats sleepwalking

Charoite

Discovered in the 1940s and originating from an area of Siberia once associated with political prisoners, charoite provided comfort and became a symbol of endurance. It is named after the Chara River in eastern Siberia, the only place in the world where it is found.

BENEFITS:

Grounds heightened spiritual energy

— Provides connection for those who work away from home or live alone with little outside contact

— Provides emotional support for those suffering from loneliness

— Talisman for acceptance and eases fears of poor health, pain, and dying

— Opens one up to their full potential and encourages service to others

— Enhances one's generosity and understanding of dualities

— Allows one to examine deeply rooted fears and determine what is real and what has been created by the mind

— Allows one to release compulsions and obsessions and calms frustration and worry

— Provides a gateway to universal energy

— Cleanses the aura and fills chakra with emotional purity

Amethyst

Derived from the ancient Greek word *amethustos*, meaning "not drunk," amethyst was carved by the Greeks into ancient drinking gourds to ward off drunkenness. It has been called the "couple's stone," as it deepens relationships and allows for a more spiritual communion.

BENEFITS:

Boosts hormone production

— Highlights root causes behind negative behaviors and emotional patterns

— Sustains peaceful energy to help one overcome addictions

— Provides comfort to those grieving the loss of a loved one

— Releases sorrow and provides understanding of the soul's eternal existence

— Carries high spiritual energy and encourages devotion to the divine

— Enhances intuition and psychic powers, including lucid dreaming

— Eliminates impatience and promotes calm and peace

— Inspires spiritual growth and enlightenment

— Protects against psychic attacks and opens channels for telepathy, clairaudience, clairvoyance, and other gifts

— Purifies the aura of negative energy and provides emotional stability

Clear Quartz

Eighth-century BCE Greek priest Onomacritus once said that anyone entering a temple with a quartz crystal in hand was certain to have his prayers answered, as the Gods could not resist its power. Today we call it the master healer stone, and it represents the largest, most diverse family in the mineral kingdom. Clear quartz contains a prismatic quality that vibrates its energy throughout all color frequencies. One must feel deserving and in harmony to receive the gifts of this crystal.

BENEFITS:

Opens the head and heart to higher guidance and allows for source energy to be translated to the physical world

— Can aid in manifestation, meditation, expanding consciousness, communication with guides, past-life recall, and attracting love by amplifying one's intention or energy

— Protects the aura and dispels static electricity to cancel out the effects of radiation

— Conducive to sleep and deciphering messages received during a dream state

— Harmonizes with the entire chakra system and demonstrates our ability to do the same

— Links the physical dimension with the spiritual

— Enhances communication with plants, crystals, animals, and higher realms

— Integrates light and positive energy into one's daily thoughts, feelings, and actions

— Increases awareness and clarity in thought

— Filters against negativity and encourages one to be mindful with their words

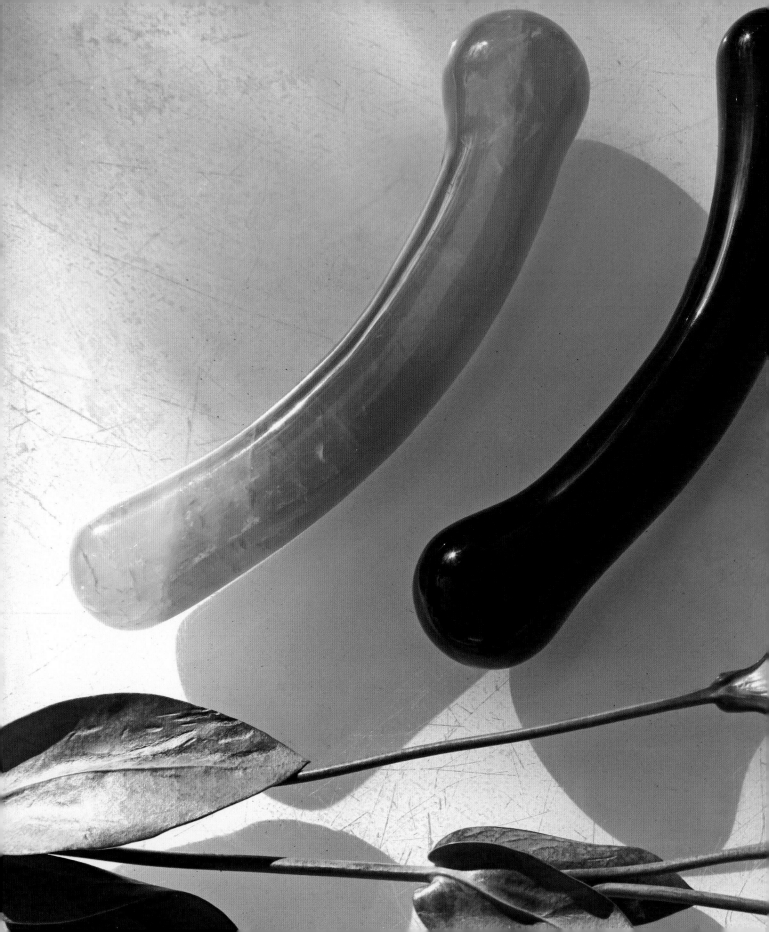

13 | OTHER METHODS OF SELF-LOVE

There are many ways of utilizing crystals to facilitate self-love and positive energy flow in your body. Once you have strengthened your connection to yourself and to the subtle vibrations of crystals, you can feel empowered to create your own exercises and rituals customized to your needs. The following are some of my favorites.

Crystal Elixirs and Massage Oils

A crystal elixir is created by infusing the energetic qualities of a specific crystal with filtered water. This allows the water to absorb the crystal's vibratory energy for storage or enhancement. When the water interacts with another life force, the energetic patterns within the crystals are manifested. This can be done by anointing yourself with the crystal elixir, watering plants with it, or drinking it.

The ancient Chinese created crystal elixirs with jade, cinnabar, and hematite for longevity, and the famous "Tan Chin Yao Ch'eh" text from approximately 600 CE discusses using mercury, sulfur, and other precious stones in elixirs. Indian Vedic texts dating back to 3000 BCE speak of elixirs as well, and powdered gemstones were used to treat a host of ailments in ancient Greece and medieval Europe. These practices have been passed down to current day; mineral salts, tinctures, and vitamin compounds are still used for their numerous healing benefits.

When choosing a crystal to create an elixir, make sure that it is non-toxic. It is safest to use an indirect, non-water-soluble method if you are unsure. Rose quartz, amethyst, and clear quartz are considered safe for mixing directly into your elixirs.

You can also create your own oil-based elixir to create crystal-infused body massage oils. Natural, organic carrier oils should be used as a base for oil elixirs. For lighter oils, charging will take a minimum of 12 hours, and for heavier oils it can take up to 28 days.

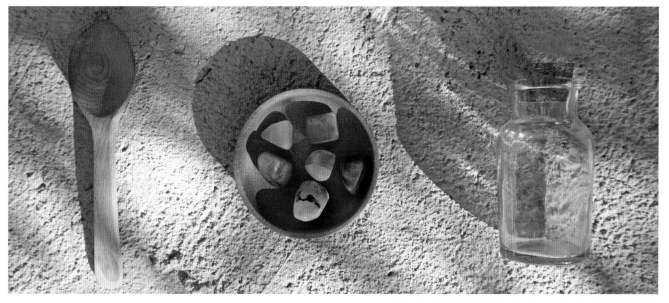

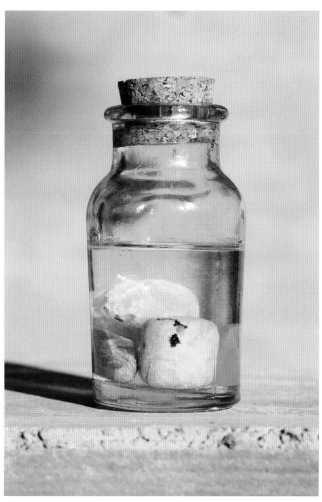

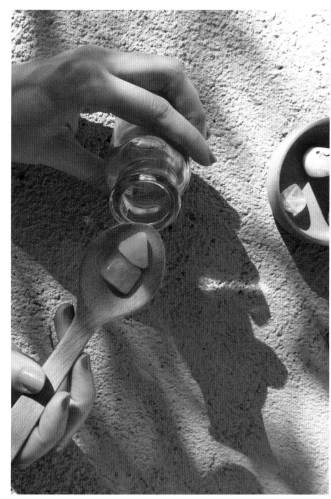

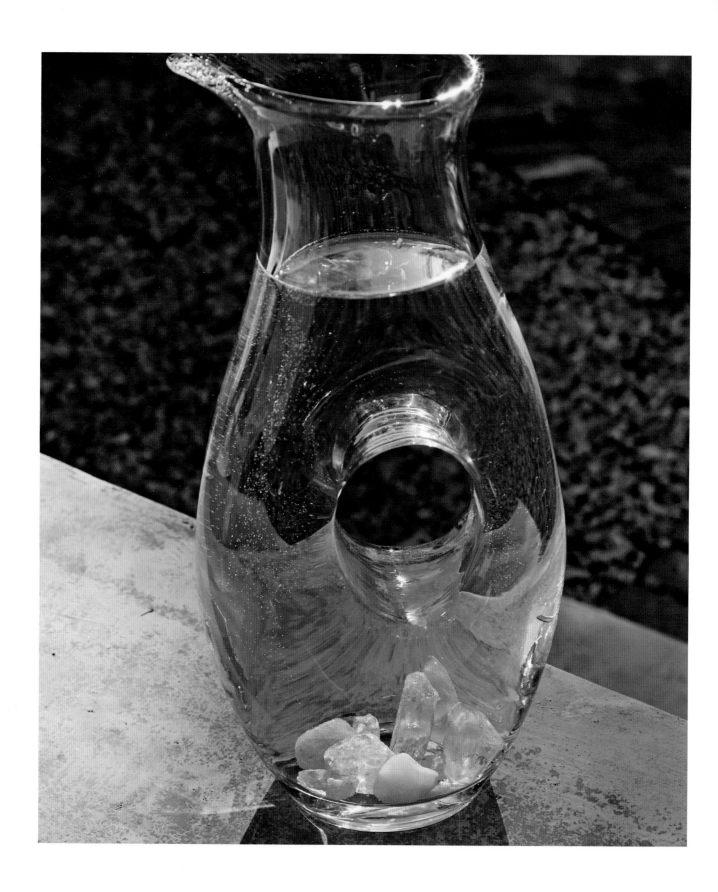

For the direct method, if using non-toxic crystals:

1. Fill a sterilized bottle with base oil.

2. Using a wooden spoon, place one cleansed stone in the oil.

3. Fasten a piece of cheesecloth over the opening of the bottle with an elastic band.

4. Place the glass bottle in the sun or in a window that gets direct sunlight to charge it.

5. Once the elixir is charged, use a clean wooden spoon to remove the stone. Add 4 to 6 drops of vegetable glycerin per 2 cups of oil to maintain the sterility of the elixir. Place the crystal in direct sunlight for several hours to re-energize it after adding the glycerin.

6. Refrigerate the elixir when not in use. It will last for up to two weeks.

For the indirect method, you'll separate the crystals with a glass barrier. This is considered the safer method, so be sure to use it if you're unsure whether the crystals you're using are non-toxic.

1. Find a drinking glass that will fit inside a glass bowl. It shouldn't be too much taller than the bowl, if at all. Using a wooden spoon, gently place a cleansed stone in the drinking glass, and place the glass in the bowl.

2. Fill the bowl with your chosen liquid to about halfway up the outside of the glass.

3. Drape a large piece of cheesecloth over the glass and bowl, securing it with a large rubber band.

4. Place the glass bottle in the sun or in a window that gets direct sunlight to charge it.

5. Remove the drinking glass and stone. Add 4 to 6 drops of vegetable glycerin per 2 cups of oil to sterilize the crystal's vibration. Alternatively, you can place the crystal in direct sunlight for several hours to re-energize it after adding the glycerin.

6. Transfer elixir from the bowl to a container with a lid before storing. Refrigerate the elixir when not in use. It will last for up to two weeks.

Chakra Foot Massage

The chakra centers in the feet are often forgotten in favor of the seven main chakras along our spine, but balancing these chakras can help stimulate and heal the entire chakra system. Anytime you feel that you need a complete energy tune-up, or just want to feel the benefits of a lovely foot massage, try this exercise, which can be done by applying pressure to the base of the feet with a charged crystal. This massage can also be done to the legs, face, and hands.

1. Take a small amount of crystal elixir (see pages 188 through 191) and warm it between your hands. Apply it to the soles and tops of your feet.

2. Using a crystal wand, apply pressure with one end of the wand at the bottom of one foot. Hold pressure firmly for about eight seconds and release.

3. Move up to the next chakra point of the foot and repeat.

4. Once you have activated each of the chakra points through pressure, repeat on the other foot.

5. Turn the wand so it is horizontal and roll it up each foot, three times each, with as much pressure as you like.

6. Move to the tops of the feet, easing the pressure of the crystal as you move over your joints. The small end of the wand can be put in between each toe, creating a soothing stretch.

Chakra Points

1. Root
2. Sacral
3. Solar Plexus
4. Heart
5. Throat
6. Third Eye
7. Crown

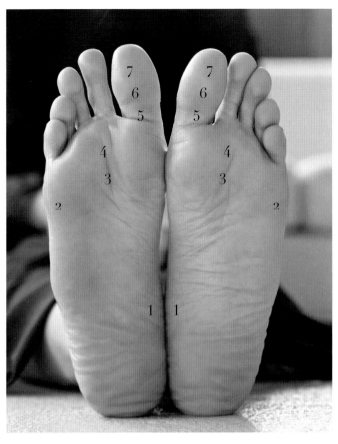

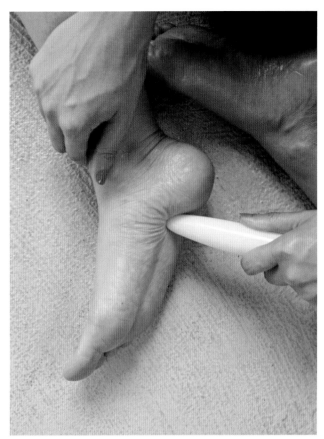

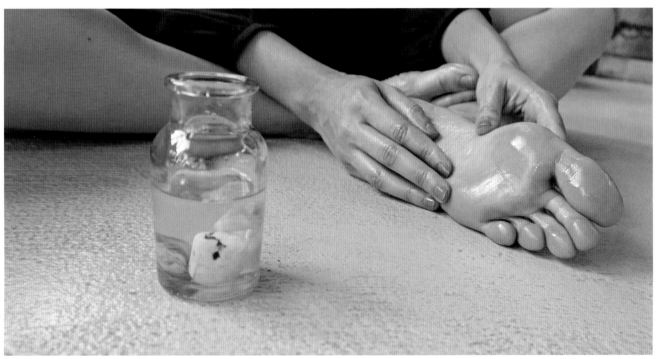

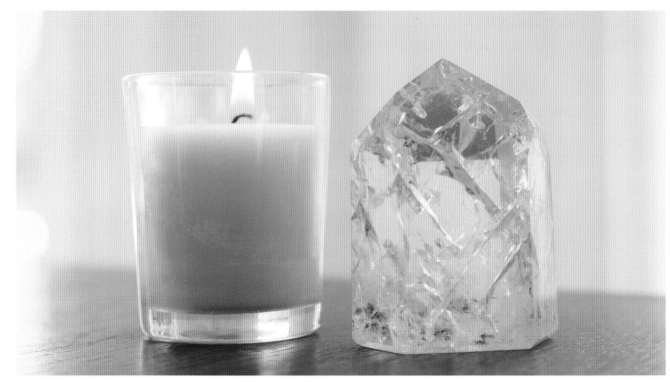

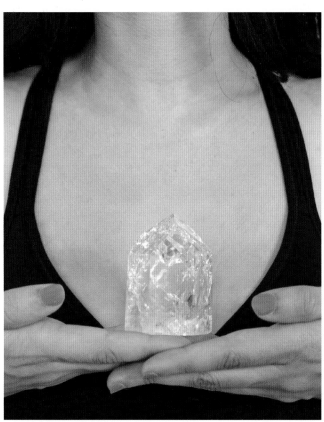

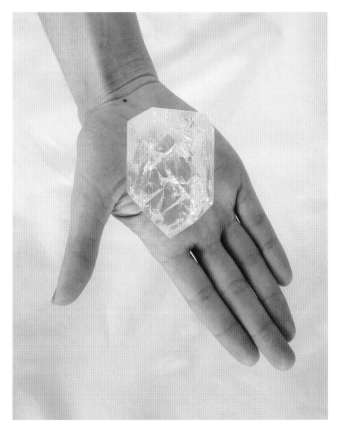

Opening the Palm Chakras

In the center of each palm are the chakras for exchanging energy. When these secondary chakras are in balance, we can give and receive, offer and accept, and so on. When we hold crystals in our palms, they empower us and connect us to the universal energy flow. Igniting energy flow in the palms allows sensual massage and touch to be taken to a therapeutic level. To open up the palm chakras, try this exercise.

1. While in a seated position, place a white quartz crystal that is small enough to fit in the palm of your hand in front of you. Light a white candle.

2. Close your eyes and breathe deeply. Do this for a few moments.

3. Rub your palms together to create warmth and hold them over the crystal. Continue to breathe.

4. Place the crystal in one of your hands, and feel its energy seeping into your palm. Direct it with your intention into your heart, creating a connection. Move the crystal to your other hand and repeat.

5. Hold the crystal in both of your hands, over your heart center. Repeat the statement, "I permit myself to feel the flow of this crystal energy through the palms of my hands. I will only give and receive energy that is beneficial and loving."

6. To seal this practice, place the crystal back in front of you and blow out the candle.

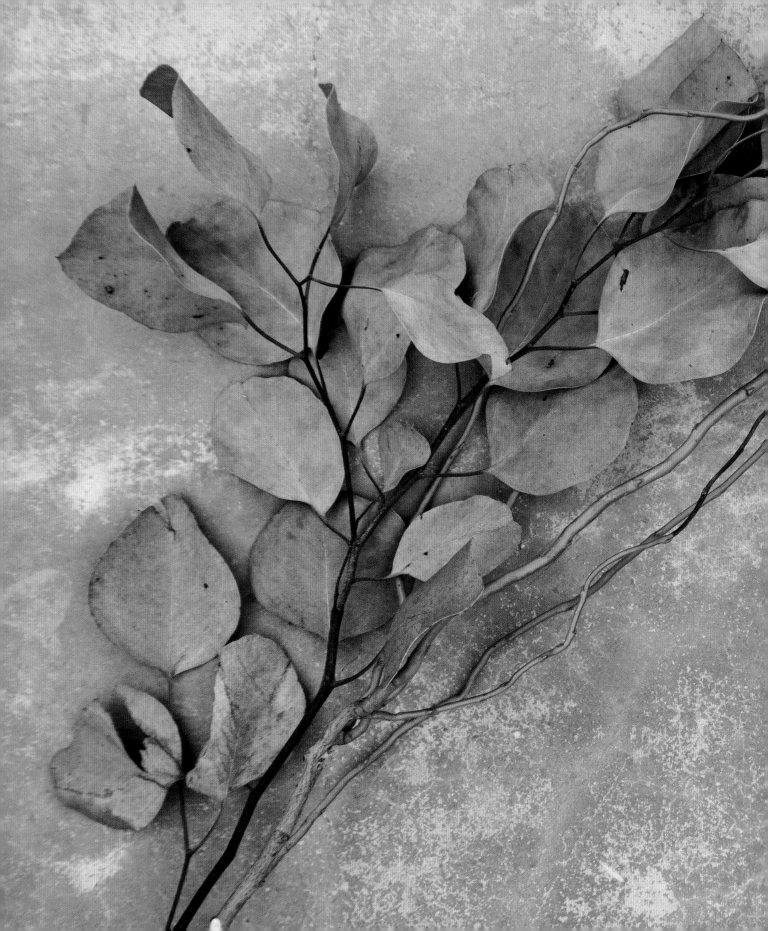

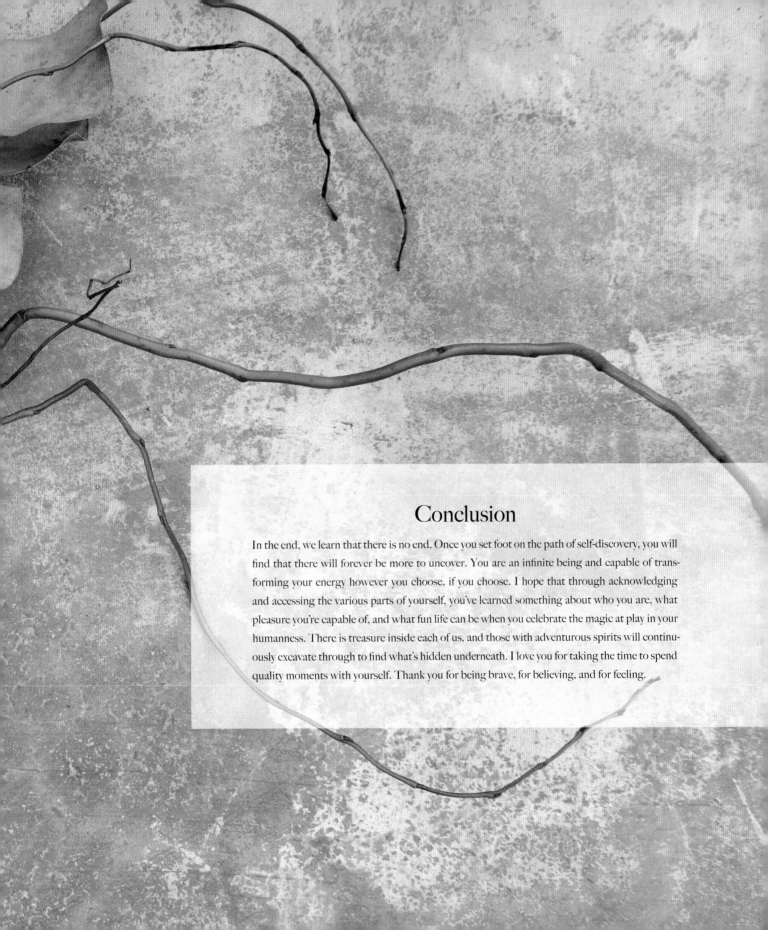

Conclusion

In the end, we learn that there is no end. Once you set foot on the path of self-discovery, you will find that there will forever be more to uncover. You are an infinite being and capable of transforming your energy however you choose, if you choose. I hope that through acknowledging and accessing the various parts of yourself, you've learned something about who you are, what pleasure you're capable of, and what fun life can be when you celebrate the magic at play in your humanness. There is treasure inside each of us, and those with adventurous spirits will continuously excavate through to find what's hidden underneath. I love you for taking the time to spend quality moments with yourself. Thank you for being brave, for believing, and for feeling.

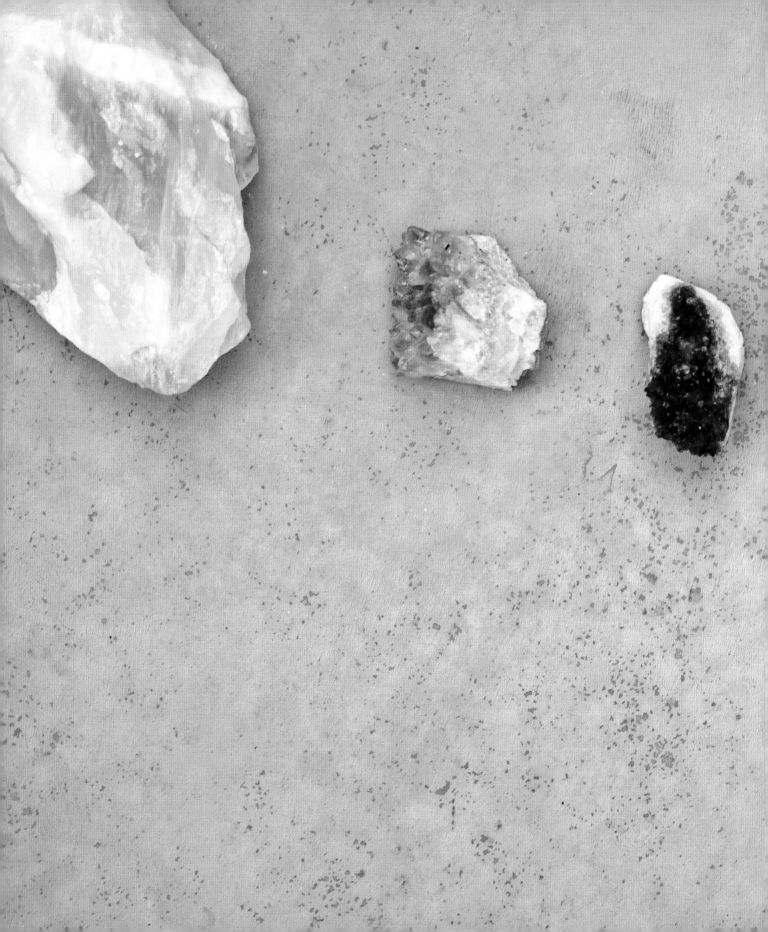

Appendices

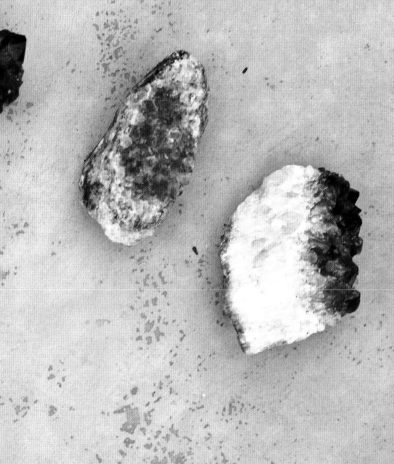
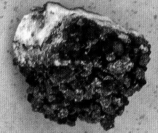

Crystals for Specific Needs

Crystals	Chakra	Zodiac	Element	Color Energy
Agate	Depending on Color	Gemini, All depending on color	Depending on color	Depending on color
Amazonite	Heart, Throat	None	Water	Turquoise
Amber	Sacral, Solar Plexus	Taurus	Water	Yellow, Gold
Amethyst	Third Eye, Crown	Aquarius	Air, Water	Violet
Apatite (Yellow)	Sacral, Solar Plexus	None	Fire	Yellow, Gold
Aquamarine	Throat	Scorpio	Water	Blue, Turquoise
Aventurine (Blue)	Throat, Third Eye	Virgo, Libra	Water	Blue
Aventurine (Green)	Heart	Virgo, Libra	Wood	Green
Aventurine (Orange)	Sacral, Solar Plexus	Taurus	Fire	Orange
Azurite	Throat, Third Eye	Sagittarius	Water	Blue, Indigo
Bloodstone	Root, Heart	Aries	Wood	Red, Green
Carnelian	Root, Sacral	Virgo	Fire	Orange, Red
Celestite	Throat, Third Eye	Gemini, Libra	Wind	Blue
Charoite	Heart, Crown	Scorpio, Sagittarius	Fire	Violet
Citrine	Sacral, Solar Plexus, Crown	Cancer	Fire	Yellow, Orange, Gold
Clear Quartz	Crown, All	All	All	White
Dumortierite	Throat, Third Eye, Crown	Leo, Virgo	Earth	Blue, Indigo
Elemental Sulfur	Solar Plexus	Leo	Fire	Yellow
Fluorite	Heart, Third Eye	Pisces	Wood	Green
Garnet	Root, Crown	Aquarius	Fire	Red, Brown
Golden Topaz	Solar Plexus	Sagittarius	Fire	Gold
Iolite	Third Eye, Crown	None	Water	Violet, Indigo

Physical Benefits

Benefits mental functioning, including concentration and analytic skills.

Beneficial for the treatment of sexual disorders such as vaginitis and priapism; balances libido.

Increases energy; relieves depression and anxiety.

Calms anxiety and nervous system; boosts hormone production.

Supports healthy appetite, posture; beneficial for teeth, bones, cartilage, and joint issues.

Respiratory and throat issues.

Calms hyperactivity; balances hormones; improves focus.

Supports cardiac and circulatory health; enhances effectiveness of homeopathic treatments.

Acknowledges physical pain brought on by sexual traumas to allow healing to occur.

Beneficial for spinal health, oxygenating blood.

Promotes hormonal balance; assists the birthing process, PMS, menstrual issues, menopause.

Supports detoxing from alcohol and drugs; invites arousal; improves circulation, lower back issues.

Relaxes tense muscles.

Supports those with ADHD; promotes restful sleep; relieves menstrual cramps.

Promotes physical stamina; aids digestion; relieves allergic reactions caused by food and chemical intolerances.

General healing.

Eases issues with the stomach, insomnia, compulsive disorders.

Helpful for skin conditions like acne and psoriasis; detoxing.

Supports teeth, bones, mental disorders.

Helps the body integrate vitamins and minerals; increases libido.

Improves brain function; alleviates nervousness.

Supports nerve function; aids digestion; improves memory.

Emotional/Spiritual Benefits

Beneficial for those healing from traumatic experiences; encourages self-acceptance.

Quells worries and aggressive behaviors; brings emotional stability and encourages healthy boundaries.

Brings about the ability to discern messages from past mistakes, transmuting them into strengths to use to manifest dreams.

Quiets the mind to better receive messages from higher realms of consciousness; releases one's addictive behaviors.

Promotes positivity, optimistic outlook; connects one to Divine Will.

Alleviates fear of the unknown; cools aggressive tendencies.

Enhances self-control; brings inner-peace; encourages creative flow.

Brings feelings of light-heartedness; allows one to see the opportunities that arise with every situation.

Calms the inner-critic, promoting love for one's own creativity.

Helps overcome the need to be a people-pleaser and in situations of being bullied.

Alleviates abandonment issues by fostering a connection to higher powers; grounding, protective.

Invigorates love for life; dispels fears of death; calms sexually related anxieties.

Gently opens one up to other dimensions; brings harmony to logic and intuition.

Gently nudges one forward through life and relationships when there is a fear of change.

Releases thought patterns that keep us in a mindset of lack; promotes feelings of abundance.

Encourages clear thinking and positive perceptions of the world.

Assists with breaking free of emotional contracts that no longer support life's journey to reach full potential.

Purifies thoughts; protects one from psychic harm.

Encourages the discernment of one's feelings in order to not act impulsively or make fear-based decisions.

Encourages desire through letting go of ingrained beliefs that inhibit self-esteem.

Assists in focusing energy to achieve one's desires; attracts the right people through enhancing one's charismatic traits and giving off an "open" vibe.

Strengthens bonds with family; brings clear solutions to difficult problems.

continued

Crystals	Chakra	Zodiac	Element	Color Energy
Jade (Nephrite)	Heart	Taurus, Libra	Wood	Green
Jasper (Red)	Root	None	Fire	Red
Kyanite (Blue)	Throat, Third Eye	None	Water	Blue
Labradorite	Throat	None	Water	Blue
Lapis Lazuli	Throat, Third Eye	Sagittarius	Water	Blue
Malachite	Heart	Taurus	Wood	Green
Menalite	Earth Star, Sacral	Cancer	Earth	White, Gray
Moldavite	Heart, Third Eye, Crown	All	Wood	Green
Moonstone	Crown	Cancer	Metal	White
Obsidian (Black)	Root	Capricorn	Water	Black
Onyx (Black)	Root	Leo	Water	Black
Pink Beryl	Heart	Taurus	Fire	Pink
Pyrite	Sacral, Solar Plexus	None	Earth	Gold
Rhodonite	Heart	None	Fire	Red, Pink, Black
Rose Quartz	Heart	Scorpio	Fire	Pink
Ruby	Root	Capricorn	Fire	Red
Sapphire (Blue)	Throat, Third Eye	Taurus	Wind	Blue
Selenite	Crown	Taurus	Water	White
Serpentine	Heart, All	Gemini	Wood, Earth	Green
Sodalite	Throat, Third Eye	Sagittarius	Water, Air	Blue
Sunstone	Root, Sacral	Leo	Fire	Gold, Orange, Red
Tiger's Eye	Root, Sacral, Solar Plexus	Gemini	Fire	Gold, Brown
Tourmaline (Black)	Root	Libra	Water	Black

Physical Benefits

Aides elimination organs; generally cleansing.

Supports childbirth, fertility, libido, and blood flow.

Relieves stress.

Respiratory issues; PMS; reduces sensitivity to cold weather.

Migraines, menstrual irregularities, issues regarding the throat.

Regulates menstrual cycle; alleviates cramps; eases labor; helps with sexual dis-ease.

Supports lactation, menopause.

Decelerates the aging process; brings clear diagnosis.

Promotes natural rhythms in the body, circadian, menstrual.

Aides in the understanding of the underlying emotional causes of physical pains.

Fortifies immune system; helps anchor excessive energy.

Valuable to support treatments for impotence and vertigo and general heart health.

Male impotence and fertility, general well-being.

Restores energy that has been drained due to emotional strain.

Softens complexion; promotes heart health; supports with postpartum depression.

Improves circulation; helps release emotional eating habits.

Insomnia, dementia, eyesight, headaches.

Energetically aligns the spine.

Relieves menstrual, muscular pain.

Cleansing for the lymphatic system; beneficial for hoarseness.

Boosts self-healing powers; relieves stomach cramps.

Decreases chance for nightmares; helps with stomach issues and disorders of the eyes.

Helps relieve body of environmental pollutants as well as "electromagnetic smog" from Wi-Fi and other electrical equipment.

Emotional/Spiritual Benefits

Brings harmony to dysfunctional relationships; facilitates strength of character.

Invigorates confidence and courage; supports those healing from verbal, emotional, and sexual abuse; Kundalini awakener.

Helps the shift of victim mentality; helps to become aware of one's natural gifts.

Enhances imagination, bringing joy through new ideas.

Empowers one through self-awareness; helps reveal the truth.

Encourages being open about one's feelings; opens one up to take risks of the heart.

Brings understanding of one's inner goddess by seeing the beauty in every phase of life.

Unites the head and the heart; inspires creative solutions.

Enhances intuition; brings a sense of ease within any environment.

Helps recognize repressed aspects of oneself in order to heal the shame that caused the repression.

Stabilizes impetuous personalities; provides energy of "self-mastery."

Aides in bringing repressed emotional needs to awareness; allows one to feel at peace when receiving compliments and love.

Diminishes fears; encourages the stamina it takes to reach one's goals.

Helps release self-destructive tendencies; promotes compassion and understanding.

Brings feelings of love in any area of life that needs it: romantic, familial, worldly, friendship.

Protects those with sensitive personalities; promotes transmutation.

Brings courage to those who feel socially awkward, encouraging self-assuredness.

Purifies inner and outer environments of negative energy.

Brings a sense of control to one's life situation.

Enhances self-acceptance; releases outdated behavioral patterns.

Helps sever ties from obsessive or possessive relationships; encourages assertiveness and the ability to say "no."

Soothes inner traumas caused by jealousy or feelings of "lack;" helps process information to improve "gut" feelings.

Purifies the mind of obsessive worries and anxieties to enable a grounded perspective.

Chakra Characteristics

Chakras	Color	Secondary Color	Musical Tone	Sensual Sound	Archetype (Positive/ Negative)	Sexuality	Location
Root	Red	Black	C	Uh	Mother/Victim	Primal, basic instincts	Base of spine
Sacral	Orange	None	D	Oo	Empress/Martyr	Giving and receiving sexual pleasure; reproduction	1 to 2 inches (3 to 5 cm) below the navel
Solar Plexus	Yellow	Gold	E	Oh	Warrior/Servant	Joyous union	Slightly to the left above the stomach
Heart	Green	Pink	F	Ah	Lover/Actor	Love	Between the breasts
Throat	Blue	None	G	I	Communicator/ Silent Child	Communication; expression	Throat
Third Eye	Indigo	None	A	Ay	Intuitive/ Intellectual	Visual/vision	Third Eye
Crown	Violet	White	B	Ee	Guru/Egoist	Spiritual experiences	Top of head

Element	Sanskrit Name	Governs	Sense	Intention	Needing Acknowledgment	Properly Functioning
Earth	Muladhara	Physical sensation, keeping you grounded, physical survival, instincts	Smell	I am	Insecure, all sexual stimulation in genitals, not-grounded, uncertain	Positive self-image, energy, stamina, confidence
Water	Svadhisthana	Relationships to others, emotions	Taste	I feel	Guilty about sex, fearful, overly-sensitive, rigidity of body and of beliefs, lack of social skills	Fluid, emotional intelligence; vital, sexual satisfaction; compassion, bonding
Fire	Manipura	Sense of personal power, fulfillment	Sight	I do	Nervousness, digestive issues	Confidence, willpower
Air	Anahata	Connection between emotional and physical love	Touch	I love	Conditional love, possessive, controlling	Compassionate, empathetic, able to surrender to sexual bliss, unconditional love
Sound	Vishuddha	Communication, expression	Hearing	I speak and am heard	Arrogant, afraid of sex, timid	Articulate, expressive, present
Light	Ajña	Intuition	No predominant sense	I see	Manipulative	Wise, master of self, charismatic
Thought	Sahasrara	Spiritual attunement	No predominant sense	I know and understand	Destructive sexual expression, depression	Spiritually connected, knowing without thought or reason

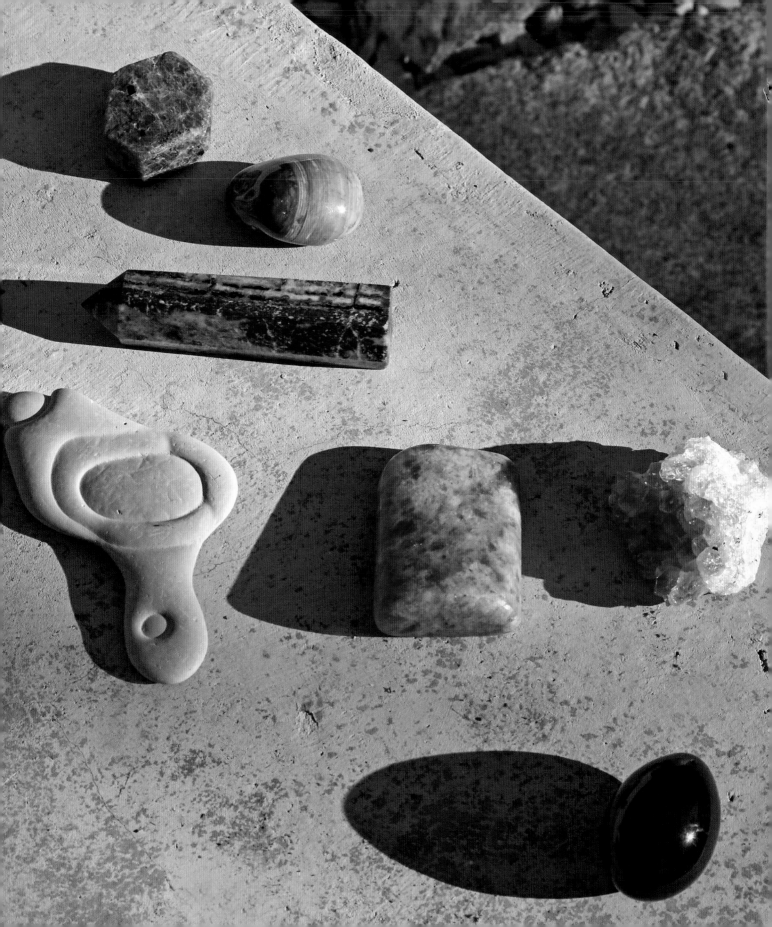

Resources

Books

The 7 Healing Chakras
  by Brenda Davies, M.D.

101 Power Crystals by Judy Hall

1911 Encyclopædia Britannica, Volume I

The Amazing Power of Deliberate Intent
  by Esther Hicks

*Amulets: Sacred Charms of Power and
  Protection* by Sheila Paine

The Art of Loving by Erich Fromm

The Boudoir Bible by Betony Vernon

The Buyer's Guide by L.S Hersh

The Complete Book of Chakras by Cyndi Dale

The Crystal Bible by Judy Hall

The Crystal Bible 2 by Judy Hall

The Crystal Bible 3 by Judy Hall

Crystal Prescriptions by Judy Hall

Crystals and Sacred Sites by Judy Hall

The Curious Lore of Precious Gemstones
  by George Frederick Kunz

Elemental Energy by Kristin Petrovich

Essentials of Geology
  by Reed Wicander and James S. Munroe

Every Dreamer's Handbook by Will Phillips

*The History & Use of Amulets, Charms and
  Talismans* by Gary R. Varner

Human Sexuality by Martha Rosenthal

Introduction to Crystallography
  by Donald Sands

Kundalini: Divine Energy, Divine Life
  by Cyndi Dale

Lucid Dreaming Plain and Simple by Robert
  Waggoner and Caroline McCready

The Metaphysical Books of Gems and Crystals
  by Florence Megemont

The Naked Woman: A Study of the Female Body
  by Desmond Morris

The New Crystal Bible by Sandra Eaton

The Path of Emotions by Synthia Andrews

Psychomagic by Alejandro Jodorowsky

Sacred Luxuries by Lise Manniche

Tao Tantric Arts for Women by Mike de Vos

Timaeus by Plato

Urban Tantra by Barbara Carrellas

Wheels of Life by Anodea Judith

Crystals

Chakrubs: The Original Crystal
Sex Toy Company
chakrubs.com

Crystal Cactus
crystalcactus.com

The Crystal Matrix
thecrystalmatrix.com

Rock Star Crystals
rockstarcrystalsmanhattan.com

Lifestyle

The Hoodwitch
thehoodwitch.com

Lola Jean
goddesslolajean.com

Naked Yoga Therapy
nakedyogatherapy.com

Sex Love Liberation
sexloveliberation.com

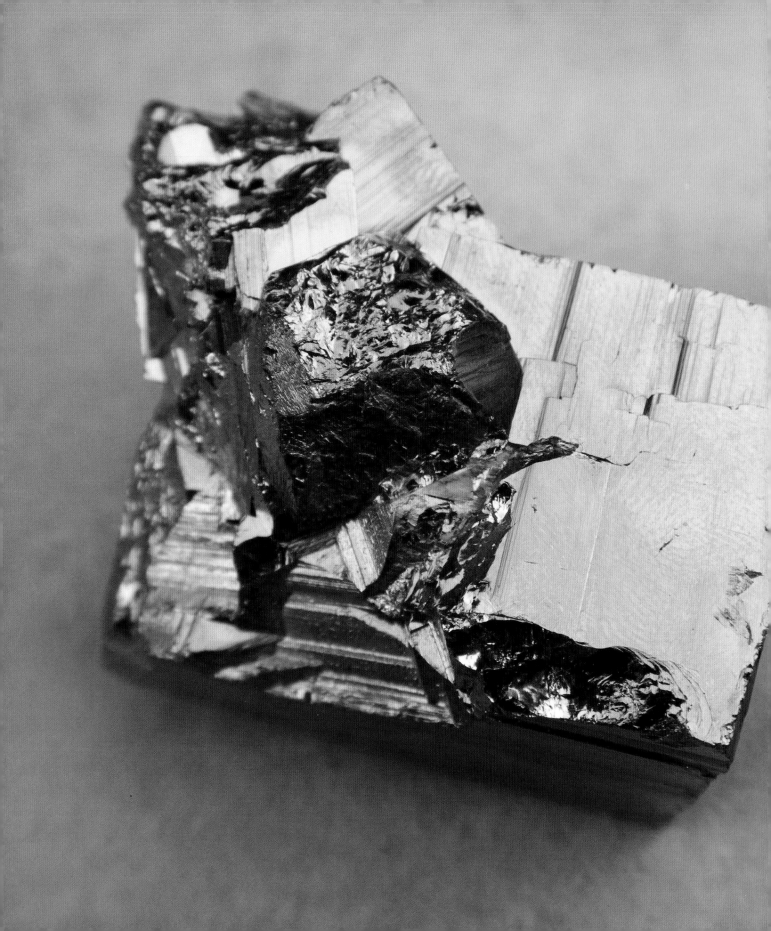

Acknowledgments

The book you hold in your hands is the collective work of many, and I am grateful to each and every one of them. To Jess Haberman and the team at Quarto for trusting my vision and taking a chance on this unique subject. To Rachel Gold for being so generous with her feedback for the rituals and beyond. To Danielle Dorsey for her tremendous support, research, and input. To Jessy Irving, for giving me peace of mind and taking care of business so I could focus on writing this book. To Kate Hollowell for capturing the beauty of the crystals in this book. To Dessi Terzieva, for not only her gorgeous styling, but the beautiful energy she brought on our adventure. To Jenny Sotelo for her dedication, organization, and creative direction. To Mom, Dad, and Marisa, for their love and support. They've all given me the tools to feel equipped to follow my dreams. And to Rachel, who is not only my sister but the only person I trusted to take my photos throughout the book. I will always be in awe of her talent and her perspective.

Finally, I'd like to take the countless people who have shared their stories and experiences with me. Thank you for being brave in acknowledging your desires and acting upon them. For giving yourself the time and attention you need. For knowing when to be gentle and when to give a push. I love you for loving yourself. Thank you.

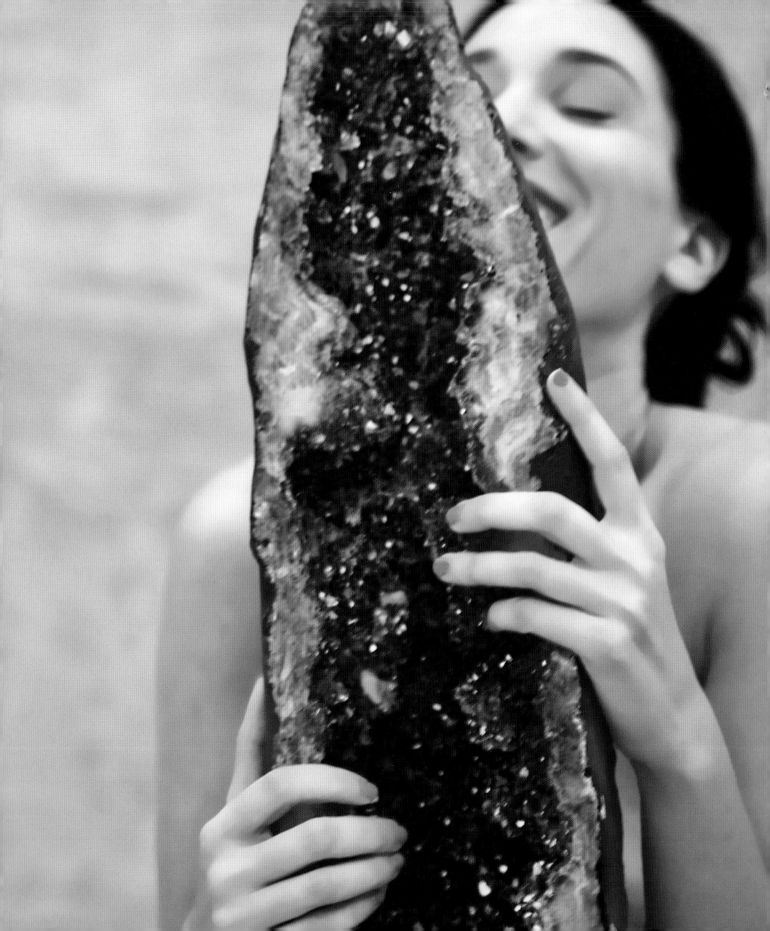

About the Author

Vanessa Cuccia is regarded as a pioneer in the sex toy industry for introducing her methods of using crystals for sexual healing and empowerment on a global scale. She is the founder and creator of Chakrubs, The Original Crystal Sex Toy Company, and she continues to receive testimonials from people around the world who use her Chakrub products and methods. These overwhelmingly positive testimonials have inspired her to write this book.

Since conceptualizing her initial designs for crystal pleasure tools in 2011 and establishing her brand in 2012, Cuccia has been an influencer in the social movement of sex positivity, self-love, and personal awareness by bridging the gap between sensuality and spirituality. As creator of products that symbolize the essence of these movements, she spearheaded the ethos of the brand which is inspiring many to nurture their own emotional intelligence, self-awareness, and spiritual connection.

Cuccia cultivated her knowledge of crystals and energy work while she was living in Los Angeles and pursuing a career in music. During this time, she worked a part-time job at an adult store where she fostered her education on sex positivity. Cuccia merged both principles, which sparked the idea of sexual exploration with the use of crystals. The recognition for the potential crystals have to facilitate energy movement inspired Cuccia to utilize crystals to enhance sexual pleasure. Cuccia's work has been a fixture in the Hammer Museum and the Museum of Sex, featured in magazines such as *New York Magazine*, *Cosmopolitan*, *Elle*, and *Allure*, appeared on notable digital platforms such as Buzzfeed and VICE, and has been featured on shows such as *The Doctors* and *Conan*. Cuccia has also received the attention of many notable artists who have collaborated with their own sensibility, bringing to light different aspects of the profound messages Chakrubs inspires.

As a certified crystal healer and reiki practitioner, Cuccia continues to pursue knowledge of crystals and metaphysical modes of healing to help those who have experienced sexual trauma or simply wish to deepen pleasure and connection to self, spirit, and others. Cuccia is a musician whose knowledge of energy extends through her performances. She currently resides in New York.

Index